A Rare Find
ETHEL AYRES BULLYMORE
Legend of an Epic Canadian Midwife

A Rare Find

Ethel Ayres Bullymore - Legend of an Epic Canadian Midwife

by Donna Mann

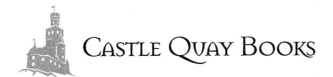

Copyright ©2013 Donna J. Mann
All rights reserved
Printed in Canada
International Standard Book Number: 978-1-927355-15-2
ISBN 978-1-927355-43-5 EPUB

Published by:
Castle Quay Books
Pickering, Ontario, L1W 1A5
Tel: (416) 573-3249
E-mail: info@castlequaybooks.com   www.castlequaybooks.com

Edited by Marina Hofman Willard and Lori MacKay
Cover design by Burst Impressions
Printed at Essence Publishing, Belleville, Ontario

This book or parts thereof may not be reproduced in any form without prior written permission of the publishers.

Library and Archives Canada Cataloguing in Publication

Mann, Donna J. (Donna Jean), 1939-, author
    A rare find : Ethel Ayres Bullymore— legend of an epic Canadian midwife / Donna Mann, Marina Hofman.
ISBN 978-1-927355-15-2 (pbk.)

    1. Kemp, Ethel. 2. Midwives—Alberta—Biography 3. Edgerton (Alta.)—Biography. I. Hofman, Marina H., author II. Title.
RG950.K44M35 2013   618.20092   C2013-905454-5

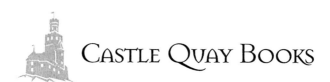

Contents

Acknowledgements 7

PART I – 1910
1. June 1910, England – The Long Night 11
2. Doctor's Orders 17
3. Looking Ahead 25
4. Grief in Goodbye 35
5. Watching Life Change 39
6. Settling In 45
7. One Step After Another 51

PART II – 1911
8. Firming Up Their New Life 59
9. Bittersweet 63
10. Time Moves On 75

PART III – 1917–1920
11. The People Find Ethel 91
12. Ethel: Prairie Nurse 99
13. Awakened to Need 105
14. Bad News–Good News 111
15. Picking Up the Pace 117
16. Perfect Timing 125
17. Slowing Down 133
18. Different-sized Gifts 137
19. The Town Gathers 143
20. Celebration in the Midst of Life 147
21. Ethel's Surprise 151
22. Double Delights 157
23. Love Finds Its Own 161

PART IV – 1921
24. Elsie Comes Home 173

Acknowledgements

As always in a long work such as this historical novel, there are many people to remember who contributed through information, reading, editing and encouragement. Thank you to Ethel's family who stood in vigil at different times over this writing: Gordon Bullymore, Debbie Sinclair-Lumme (Bullymore), Russell Umbach, Margo Umbach, Nikki Markwart, and Sandra Taylor. Thank you to friends of the Bullymore family, who wrote letters, sent pictures and placed phone calls. A special thanks to Eadie Buchanan, Mary Walker and Erica Bonner Cooper who opened many doors of memory.

In the early days of writing, during my visits to England and in prolonged research, my historian cousin, Robin Harris, guided me through many geographical locations. As well, Canadian and British archivists and researchers were very helpful. Early readers such as Bonnie Mallard, N.J. Lindquist, Karen Stiller, Bridget Forester, Maxine Hancock, Angelina Fast-Vlaar, Ruth and Tom Sproule, Rosemary Tanner, Pat Mestern, Ray and Anna Wiseman, and Wanda who, in the midst of her grief, sympathized with Ethel's sorrow and celebration, assisted and encouraged me.

Thank you to those friends, especially the registered nurses, who defined and refined medical terms into everyday language: Marion Israel, Bette Speer, Rose Anne Kreps, Sharron Howse-Mann and Grace Ann Gibson.

I'm continually encouraged through The Word Writers, Word Weavers, The Word Guild and Write! Canada. Thank you to my husband, Doug, who probably read this manuscript a dozen times and still appreciated the story. A word of gratitude to Larry Willard (Castle Quay Books Canada) for believing in this story, always keeping in touch at the right moments, and finally saying, "Yes, we'll publish this." And to Marina Hofman Willard who coached the manuscript from labour pains through to birth.

PART I
1910

chapter one

June 1910, England – The Long Night

Brushing her fingers against the small envelope tucked inside her skirt pocket, Ethel Kemp remembered her sadness while preparing its content. She blinked the tears back, reflected on her morning prayers and straightened her shoulders. "We can do this."

The large doors of Enfield Cottage Hospital felt extra heavy as she pushed them open. As a practical nurse, she especially liked floor duty, where bonding with new mothers and babies lasted long after she left the ward. And night shift, definitely her favourite time to work, opened a world of ongoing activity that defied darkness.

The familiar sounds of clinking metal pans, women's laboured groans and the constant movement of busy nurses already provided a prelude to her night's work. Strong-smelling disinfectant infused her senses, confirming that cleanliness was next to godliness—and both were welcome on this floor.

"It doesn't seem to matter what you begin in life, ladies, the pain of letting go and the hope of new beginnings go hand in hand," Ethel murmured as she walked toward the medical ward, familiar to her as Mum's kitchen. Goodness, she'd experienced enough of both in her own life to know this personally!

Looking at the large wall clock as she entered the hospital change room, she grinned—Nurse Rankin was up to her old tricks, 10 minutes fast. *Have to love that woman; she looks after us—one way or the other.* Ethel tucked a curl under her cap, glad she'd taken time to pin her dark unruly hair tightly into a bun. With her starched apron covering her uniform, she gave a last-minute check to her gleaming white oxford shoes.

Nurse Rankin was particular about the appearance of her staff, boasting that their personal care and presentation to the public gave a clear message about her nurses. There was no room for anything less than absolute correctness, and Ethel felt privileged to work under her professional competence.

Even though she wished Nurse Rankin had a sense of humour to lessen the stress that regularly shrouded their work, she definitely offered a professional presence that greatly influenced Ethel: a calming authority in times of life and death situations. And last night, there was more death than life on this ward.

The room smelled fresh as Ethel filled the small sink with hot water. She added the disinfectant soap and then quickly finished the routine task of scrubbing her hands. As the green suds ran down the drain, she thought how quickly life could change with just one action.

She sat down a few minutes later at the nurses' desk and greeted Nurse Rankin. While listening to report, Ethel learned that a sick baby and a new mother had kept the staff busy on the previous shift. Two women laboured now, one bleeding enough to keep the doctor and the other practical nurse by her bedside, while her family waited in the lobby.

The younger of the two women, Rosie, had come in alone, and she'd leave alone; her baby was going to the orphanage. Ethel wondered about the girl's heartache and was glad she'd come to the hospital when her labour had developed problems, rather than giving herself over to some blundering, wine-guzzling hussy in the dirty bedroom of a back alley flat.

Rosie's cries cut through the dimness. "Can 'e come, ma'am? Can 'e come—now? Oh, God help, me baby's coming."

Ethel took long strides across the softly lit room while the shadow of her hourglass figure played along the wall. She looked down at the watch glistening against her bib, and then gently lifted it to see the time to chart later. Even in this moment of concern, she remembered her graduation day and the thrill of her father pinning on the watch.

She pulled the curtain back, adjusted the light and picked up a crumpled pillow lying on the floor. The cotton cover lay strewn to one side as Rosie's body writhed in pain, her arms and legs thin as the wooden stick-dolls Pa carved.

"Miss Rosie," Ethel said softly, standing beside her bed. "How are you, now?"

"The pains keep coming, but nothing happens."

Rosie's fine features, pale from stress and pain, reminded Ethel of a weathered porcelain doll.

"Just a little while yet," Ethel said, as she put a cold cloth on Rosie's forehead. "Don't be afraid of your pains. You're getting closer. Every pain helps your little one further along. Breathe deeply and try to relax."

June 1910, England – The Long Night

Ethel wondered about Rosie's family. That poor girl had been working away since yesterday morning without help, alone with her fears and pain. *Pity, it is— these young ones having to go through this alone. Everybody should have a friend or family waiting.*

"Do you have the name of a family member if we should need to call anyone?"

"No, I don't, ma'am. My ma don't want to know, and if my pa know'd, he'd kill me. And, well, I can't tell the one who ought'a know."

"I'm sorry," Ethel said, remembering her own loneliness in Tom's absence when their daughter Elsie was born. "It's a lonely time, isn't it? Just hold on. In a few hours, this'll be all over. Try to think on that."

"Thank you, ma'am. I like the sound of your voice. I think if God had a voice, it might sound something like yours."

"I'm sure God has a voice, and maybe you're hearing it in your heart. And it's telling you that you're out of harm's way." Ethel straightened the pillow under Rosie's head and thought of the grief that must fill her heart at this time when she should be able to look forward to happiness with her child.

Ethel never took labour pains and deliveries for granted; nor did she ever make light of them. They amazed her as she waited for a new life to slide into the world and announce its arrival with loud wailing.

Rosie's baby girl had done just that, an hour after Ethel had taken that few minutes to encourage her.

As the night turned to morning, quietness lingered like a comfortable blanket. Ethel enjoyed the silence and the sense that her mums and babes had settled. Charts completed and filed, waiting for the next shift, gave Ethel satisfaction. It would be difficult to say goodbye to all of this, but she must do it.

At the end of her shift, Ethel left the ward and stood at the back hall window. Foggy morning light that framed the smoke-stained buildings across the alley limited her view. She looked down at the soot and dust on the exterior windowsill and shook her head as if to clear her mind to think pleasant thoughts. Tom!

More than four years since she had said goodbye to her beloved, and she remembered his promises with clarity. "We'll get us married and go to Canada, luv, you 'n me, and we'll make a new beginning." But it hadn't happened. Between health issues and family upheavals, they'd never managed their dream. The doctor had told him repeatedly, "Your breathing's getting worse, Tom. If you don't soon go, you might have difficulty getting through immigration."

Twice they'd made their plans and postponed their trip, but in 1906, due to his poor health, Tom had finally left for Alberta, Canada without her. Ethel had cried for weeks. It wasn't long before she began to think she might never see him again—and that he might never see their unborn child.

"Tired, Nurse?" Nurse Rankin asked, coming up behind her.

"Yes, ma'am," Ethel answered. "I'm always tired after working nights. I'll sleep like a baby when I go home." Ethel paused, and then put her hand in her pocket and pulled out the envelope. "Nurse Rankin, I was going to come to your office, but since you're here, I'll speak to you now if that's permissible."

Nodding, she said, "Yes, of course. What is it?"

"There's something I have to do that gives me great distress." Ethel slowly handed the sealed paper to her.

Nurse Rankin opened it, read the words and then looked at Ethel. "Moving to Canada, are you?" She looked back at the letter. "It's a big step. Are you ready for such a change?"

"I wonder if I'll ever be ready." Ethel frowned. "There's times when I think it'd be easier to just stay put." She looked out the window again. "When I gave up my flat, I think it made everything real. It was the beginning of leaving so much behind." She dropped her voice to almost a whisper. "It's been hard coming to this decision for many reasons. My father is not at all well, and—"

"Is it something you have to do?"

"Yes, ma'am. I've been thinking about it for a long while. My Tom's breathing got so bad, he had to go on without me. In his last letter, he said that he'd takin' to fits of coughing, again. There's been so many things that's kept Elsie and me from joining him, the last one being her bout of scarlet fever. For a while, I thought we'd never be able to make the trip. However, I decided if I don't go soon, it might be too late. I've been saving, so I purchased tickets for Elsie and me. And, well, we think the time is right."

"I'm sorry it's been so difficult for you, Miss Kemp," Nurse Rankin said. "I had no idea." She folded the letter. "I cannot imagine your pain. I know how you love working here and how important your family is to you."

"Yes, ma'am. There are times when I don't think I can leave all of this." Ethel grimaced, looking past Nurse Rankin. She stepped closer and began again. "But now it's all decided, and yesterday, the post brought confirmation that we leave Liverpool on July 7th, aboard the SS *Lake Manitoba*, an immigrant ship." A sob of joy caught in her throat at the thought of her and Elsie spending Christmas with Tom.

June 1910, England – The Long Night

Ethel and Nurse Rankin both stood silent, as if waiting for the other one to speak.

"I'm really sorry to lose you, lass. Write to me when you need a reference."

"Thank you." Ethel pulled a tissue from her pocket and wiped a tear from her cheek. "You've been very good to me. I'll miss you."

"And that feeling is mutual. You bring a love to this floor as I've never experienced in forty years of nursing." Nurse Rankin chuckled. "I have to admit, though, I've feared at times that you'd end up taking all the hurting ones home with you."

"I know," Ethel said as she slowly opened her hands and laced her fingers together. "It's not that I haven't thought about it. And thank you, ma'am, for your kind words. I've enjoyed working here, and I'll miss all of you."

"You know, lass, I think you'll do fine." Nurse Rankin touched Ethel's shoulder and lingered for a moment. "Remember those labour pains. Happens in more of life than we give credit—usually a sign of good things to come. God bless you in your new life."

Ethel thought her superior was going to hug her, but she spun around and walked away. Turning, Ethel squinted through the grime-coated window at the dull morning light. She wanted to be excited about this decision and the journey ahead, but she couldn't shake the foreboding of grief surrounding her.

chapter two

Doctor's Orders

Two weeks later, Ethel and her mother walked through the market towards the train station, picking up their skirts as they stepped across the gutters. The warm June air promised a pleasant summer day. Ethel shifted the bulky parcels under her arm and walked along the familiar street, glad she'd accepted Mum's invitation to go to the shops. They jostled forward, careful to avoid the horses that pulled their drays and buggies along the street. The chatter of the shoppers aggravated Ethel's unsettled mind. She usually loved London with its shops and crowds, but today seemed like an endurance race in which she'd lost sight of the finish line.

Suddenly, yells and screams of protest added to the clamour. Throngs of people began to gather, raising their arms, pushing and cursing.

"What's going on? What are people so angry about?" Ethel asked as she craned her neck to see.

"Well, I'm not about to go and find out," Mum said.

Ethel's curiosity piqued. "Just move over here a bit, Mum, and then we'll be out of the way. Maybe we can see what's happening."

Bobbies shoved their way into the centre of the crowd, shouting orders and threatening to use their sticks. Groups of people huddled together off to the side of the market, talking and laughing, sometimes heckling. Several people crammed in front of Ethel, forcing her to stand on tiptoe to see over their heads. Slowly, she led Mum in front of the shops, staying away from the big crowd in the middle of the market.

A lorry with high wire sides cut through the mob. A new group of bobbies jumped from it, swinging their sticks over the people's heads and shouting mocking words that caused the crowd to shrink back. The bobbies promptly dropped the tailgate. A grinding sound resonated through the air.

A man behind Ethel grumbled, "Next thing, those women'll want a seat in parliament."

Ethel's throat tightened and her heart pounded as she watched the bobbies drag some women by their hair, push and shove the rest, and throw them into the back of the lorry. They cried out, but the bobbies paid little attention to their pleas. After slamming the large doors shut, the officers climbed onto the running boards. The lorry with its passengers sped away.

Within minutes, the market had cleared of all the observers. Placards and posters with bold black letters spelling *Votes for Women* lay strewn across the dirty street.

Tears welled up in Ethel's eyes. "Oh, Mum. Those poor women! What are they guilty of—speaking their minds and wanting to have an opinion? Surely we're not that feared."

With the afternoon spent, Ethel and Mum boarded their train and rode most of the way home to Enfield in silence. As the train chugged into the Enfield station, Ethel began to gather her bags.

"I'm going back into London on Friday for Elsie's final medical appointment. I hope we don't run into that hostility again. I don't want to expose Elsie to it."

"You'll be fine, luv," Mum said. "Just keep away from the square."

Ethel knew it would take more than staying away from the square to avoid suffragists. They could appear at the most unexpected times and surprising places. Only yesterday, she'd read in the *London Times* that 153 women were arrested on Downing Street for rioting; one, an elderly woman, was in a self-propelled invalid chair. Ethel smiled, in spite of the horror of the incident. She would delight in being that woman's nurse.

The sun shone brightly when Ethel and Elsie stepped down from the train onto the London platform a few days later. Elsie, petite with long brown wavy hair held back by barrettes, attracted people with her quick smile and big eyes. Ethel couldn't help thinking that Elsie, as trusting as she was, would stand and chat with anybody, especially when she could announce she was getting new shoes.

A magician standing on a red box caught Elsie's attention. An inquisitive child by nature, she squealed with delight when he noticed her. She laughed as she watched him work wonders with his high black hat and long silver cane. He had rabbits, doves, many flags and silk scarves. He knew his trade well. A dozen or more people applauded him, and Elsie jumped with obvious excitement. A keen child with infectious laughter—Ethel enjoyed watching her.

Standing in front of a wooden street bench, Ethel brushed accumulated dust and bits of twig off the surface. Lifting her hand to wave, she remembered how well Elsie had fared through the long six weeks of scarlet fever. She'd cried with her sore throat and headache but had tolerated the rash well. Seeing her today, jumping with joy at the magician's tricks, made it easy to forget she was ever a sickly child.

"Come on. We'd better go," Ethel called, looking across the street to the big clock set into the wall of the ancient stone building.

"No! No!" Elsie shouted.

"Yes, dear," Ethel said. "Right now."

Elsie headed toward her mother. "He is so funny."

"Yes, that magician was very good," Ethel said and laughed. "I don't think I've seen such antics since I was a child. I'm glad you enjoyed the man with the balloons and funny hat, sweetheart."

"Yes, Mummy. Can the funny man come with us?" Elsie asked.

"I'm afraid not, dear. He's going to make other little girls laugh, and we need to get those new shoes before we're off to the doctor's office to hear how well you're doing."

Doctor Austin hurriedly flipped through a pile of papers in a large file as though looking for a particular one. "I'd like to take a little extra time with you, Miss Kemp, if that's possible. I'll try to be brief, but there's a few things we have to talk about."

"Oh?" Ethel looked straight at him.

"First," the doctor raised his eyebrows, "how is Tom doing?"

"In his last letter, he told me how much he enjoys his butcher shop. He did say his cough is back, but other than that, he's enjoying Canada."

The doctor sighed. "I think about him often." He frowned and put his finger to his chin. "Now for Elsie. I have the results from her last test."

At the mention of her name, Elsie came to her mother's side. With a puzzled expression, she looked up at the doctor.

Ethel took Elsie to a corner of the doctor's office, gave her some blocks to play with, and then returned to her seat. "Yes, go on." Ethel leaned forward.

"I have no doubt in my mind that the bacteria that causes scarlet fever can also initiate other conditions. Unfortunately, Elsie has developed a weak heart, and it's something we have to watch." The doctor raised a hand to prevent interruption. "This is not unusual. We knew there was a problem from Elsie's initial medical examinations, but I didn't see it as a crisis until now."

"I thought she was coming along just fine." Ethel pressed a hand to her chest, her own heart pounding fast.

"There's always caution following scarlet fever or any childhood disease, as you well know. I don't want to alarm you unduly, but now…now since my last examination, I'm certain she has a greater problem." The doctor paused. "I'm sorry, but I feel she is at risk."

"At risk? What does *at risk* mean?" Scenes of her family's sorrow fled through Ethel's mind when she remembered her older brother's death 11 years ago. The doctor had told Pa that Will had fainted and then died due to a weakened heart, probably caused from an earlier bout of influenza. He was only 16 years old, with his whole life ahead of him. Ethel caught a sob in her throat. Could that happen to Elsie? Oh, God forbid it!

"Scarlet fever can stress the kidneys and the heart." The doctor broke into her thoughts. "And we don't know a lot about why these two organs are affected more than others. But we do know that a patient who's had scarlet fever should have special care following the disease—especially a child. We have to admit, Elsie did have quite a serious bout. And we want to be sure she can lead a healthy and active life as she grows up." Shuffling his papers, the doctor continued, "You'll know all this, of course, from your nursing experience."

"Yes, I understand. But do you think that in Elsie's case it's so serious?" Ethel asked.

"I'm afraid so. I'm relieved to have had the time to determine this."

Ethel cleared her throat and rubbed her hands together as if warming them. "What are you saying? I mean, you're aware that I've arranged passage to Canada in a short time. Is there something that can be done before then?"

"No, there isn't. Well, not immediately anyway." The doctor came out from behind his desk and sat on the corner. He looked over at Elsie, then to Ethel. "What I'm going to suggest will be difficult to hear."

"Yes?" Ethel straightened her back. "Go on."

"Your family situation is very common. Individual members of a family are often sick with various conditions that need different care. Tom, for instance, needed to leave England to look after his lungs. He was still a young man with a chance to work and save for his family. But staying here with his condition, as well as continually being exposed to disease, would have limited any chance of recovery for him."

"I understand that. But what does that mean for Elsie?"

"Let me continue. You should go to Canada and get yourself settled. Elsie, on the other hand, because of her health should not go, just yet."

"No!" Ethel stood. The chair legs screeched on the linoleum floor. "I won't hear of it."

"Now, just think this through."

"No, Doctor Austin. I will not leave Elsie behind, if this is what you're suggesting. And that's final. My goodness, how could I even consider it? How could I survive being separated from her?" Ethel lowered her head. "And what would people say?"

She quickly turned away, as if to free herself from this distressing situation. Her heart raced. She wanted this conversation to stop.

Doctor Austin continued. "Perhaps you're not aware of it, but people do this all the time. I have several patients who are leaving their children in England and travelling to Canada—for various reasons. Education is, of course, a big factor, and health is as well. Perhaps if you could talk to some of these people, they'd help you understand that it isn't so terrible to want the best for your children, regardless of whether you're the one who provides it or you arrange for someone else to do so. You just do what you have to do."

Ethel looked at the doctor and swallowed. He was right, of course. A family of the neighbourhood came to mind. But not her family. There'd been enough separation. She wouldn't have it. That was final.

"This might be all right for somebody else, but my goodness, Elsie's only four years old. She needs me," Ethel pleaded.

"Yes, she does. And I'm the first to admit that being together is the ideal situation. However, we're dealing with reality. The tests show that her condition requires special monitoring. You won't have the same access to medical care as you've had here, and I feel it's crucial to examine and watch her regularly over the next few months. Also, it'll be extremely stressful for her to endure a long crossing, plus the ongoing tension of adjusting to a new environment."

"This your final word, Doctor?" Ethel asked.

"Yes. I'm afraid it is."

"Then, perhaps I should consider not going? I could—"

"I'm recommending that you go on—without Elsie for the time being. Go to Tom. You can both prepare for Elsie to join you as soon as I feel she can travel. I'll write to you and keep you informed."

As though caught in a press, Ethel struggled to breathe. Tom and Elsie were the two most important people in her life. How could she tolerate separation from either one of them? Tom in Canada and Elsie here. Wherever she was, Ethel would have to be without one of the persons she loved. She sat still and closed her eyes, as if to shut out reality. Then, she gathered her skirts, walked over to Elsie and hugged her before turning towards the door.

"Thank you, Doctor. We mustn't keep you any longer." Ethel's voice broke and she continued softly, "Should you have reason to change your mind about this, please be so kind as to inform me by post at Mum's address in Enfield."

"Very well. I'm sorry I couldn't have better news for you. But I assure you, this solution is for the best."

Ethel nodded goodbye to the doctor and then quietly directed Elsie down the dark corridor and out into the sunlight of a summer afternoon.

The day had grown humid, and the warm damp London air hung around them like a wet cover. They trudged along the crowded street.

Ethel tucked Elsie's hand into hers, feeling small fingers lace through her own. "Don't you worry none," she said to Elsie, juggling her bag and purse in her other hand, "we'll work something out, sweetheart."

"What, Mummy?"

"About what the doctor said."

"He's playing pretend," Elsie scoffed as she toddled along beside Ethel.

"We'll talk about it later, dear. Right now, we have to hurry to reach our train."

The engine sat belching steam, beyond the massive gateway. They quickly made their way up the steps and entered the carriage, Ethel clutching two return tickets in her hand. After finding a seat, she settled Elsie beside her. Elsie picked at the needlework on the cape of her navy serge box coat and tugged at her cotton bonnet, causing it to tip and release curls to fall around her freckled face. She wiggled in the seat, parted her cape and quickly straightened her neatly ironed bodice-dress. Wide eyed with a raised brow, she looked at her mother.

"I'm good today, Mummy. See? I'm better, 'n't I?" Elsie asked through tears.

"I think you are, sweetheart." Ethel put her arm around Elsie to give her a hug. "And that makes me happy." Elsie's bonnet suddenly took on the appearance of a tilted halo, and Ethel smiled.

"I'm not sick, I'm not, Mummy," Elsie said.

Doctor's Orders

"I'm glad you don't have those nasty old headaches anymore," Ethel replied. "My scarlet fever's all better."

Ethel laughed. "It's been a long time since you've been sick. Your dolly doesn't get hugged nearly as much now that you're feeling better." She drew Elsie close.

Elsie rummaged through Ethel's bag to retrieve her doll and a couple of picture books. Ethel felt her push tightly against her side as she snuggled under her arm. After a bit of time, she stretched out on the seat and went to sleep. Ethel noticed how relaxed she looked in spite of the train's noise and jostling.

The doctor's news had been harsh. It was just unthinkable. She simply couldn't bear it. Tears streamed down her cheeks. She reached over and pushed a moist lock of hair from Elsie's brow.

"I can't think of life without you, Elsie," Ethel whispered as she rested her head back against the seat. She'd be sad to leave the family, but now Elsie…it was too much. Sobs rose in her throat and she swallowed them back. Oh God, how could she do this?

Tom's voice echoed, "It's a chance of a lifetime…I mean, to go to Canada with the opportunity for jobs. Everything I've read boasts a land of plenty. Their printed posters say it's a perfect place to live, with plenty of land for everybody and a chance to make a good life."

Ethel said softly, "But, without you, Elsie, how can we even enjoy any of that? It'd be like leaving a piece of ourselves back here."

That's exactly what she would be doing, and it grieved her. She sighed and longed for the quietness of her church. More than anything else now, she needed to sit in her familiar pew and ask God to help her accept this decision and do the impossible.

chapter three

Looking Ahead

"Mum, I have to talk to you." Ethel walked into the kitchen, interrupting Elizabeth Kemp's humming as she sat at the table peeling potatoes. Elsie ran to play with Evie, her little auntie.

"What is it? You're all right to travel, aren't you?"

"Yes, but…it's not me, Mum. It's Elsie. I've got bad news from the doctor." Ethel turned her head and began to sob. "She's developed a heart problem…the doctor suspects from the scarlet fever. She can't come to Canada with me."

"There, there, dear." Mum laid her potato and knife on the oilcloth-covered surface and walked over to Ethel. Wrapping her arms around Ethel, she said, "How can that be possible? Are you sure you heard him right?"

"That's what he said," Ethel said, leaning into her mum. "And he won't change his mind. He won't even consider me waiting for another year until Elsie's stronger. He says I should go now and help Tom prepare a home for all of us."

The kitchen with its familiar shiny cupboard tops and organized dishes and pans reminded Ethel of the many good meals and conversations and the love shared in this room. Today, it seemed like a haven away from the cruel choices of life.

Mum stepped back and placed wrinkled hands on her hips. "Then, my dear, that's exactly what you must do. Elsie will stay with us. Your father and I will take good care of her. It won't be forever."

Ethel looked at her mother's favourite pose. She'd seen this other times whenever Mum was serious about doing something difficult.

"It seems like it." Ethel wiped her nose with her handkerchief. "Anyway, it's just too much to ask of you, with your young ones and all. Why, you'd have both Evie and Elsie at almost the same age. That'd be enough to drive you down the road." Ethel shook her head.

"The other children can help," Mum said. "We can handle it."

"I can't bear to think of it." Ethel slumped down in a chair beside the kitchen table. "I don't know what I'd do without Elsie. And I'm so afraid. What if—"

"Now, now, enough of that," Mum said. "You've plenty to think about without the *what ifs* in life."

"You know how it hurts." Ethel wiped a tear away. "I remember like it was yesterday when our Will died with a weak heart—and him so young."

"I remember too, lass…our firstborn," Mum said. "But this is different. You'll see Elsie again." Her voice softened. "I know it won't be easy for you, but think how complicated it would be if you had to cope with Elsie's health during the crossing, and then all the settling once you arrive, never mind getting her away to school in the next year or so." She placed a loaf of bread on the table. "And you don't know how Tom's going to be when you get there."

"Tom's all right, Mum," Ethel countered. "I can tell by his letters. We'd manage." Ethel folded her handkerchief. "I just can't bear to go on without her. Maybe there'll be more organized care in Canada and—"

"Ethel, rest assured we'll work out things for Elsie right here at home. Your pa and I, we'll get along fine." Mum turned and faced Ethel. "Now Canada's another story; it's a colony. Don't count on better ways. I know you're very taken with all the Canadian propaganda, but you have to realize the country isn't established like England." She leaned over and held Ethel's hand. "But we'll talk about that later. Your father is going to be home for supper, and the table won't be laid if I don't get to it." She wiped her hands on her apron. "You go wash up."

After Mum cleared the supper dishes, Pa and the younger children played on the floor in front of the cook-stove. "Come on, lass," she said, "sit down and have your tea. I think we'd better talk about Canada, a wee bit." She put the teapot on the table. "There are lots of things you will find the same over there. For instance, a church will be as important to you in Canada as it has been here. Friends will be a grand support for you. Family will be of the utmost importance. Learning about life in general will hold as many surprises as it did for you here. And that's only a few similarities. But, there's another side that you will discover." Mum picked up the salt and pepper shakers and placed them on the cupboard shelf. "I've read about Canada being the *Wild West*, a frontier land. Guns, bears, Indians, buffaloes and tar-paper, even sod houses. It sounds like another world."

"I know, I've read that too," Ethel said. "But I don't think that's Edmonton."

"Edmonton's a young city, still developing in many ways. You're not going to find the shops and fashions like you see in London. The variety of food and available supplies for your family may be quite different, as well as medical resources and information. You have to realize you'll be stepping into a completely new situation."

"In spite of all that, Tom and I could cope with Elsie's condition," Ethel argued.

"I don't doubt that for a minute, luv, but you have to get used to the fact that Edmonton won't be like here. You'll see lots of poverty, sickness and violence over there."

"I've seen all that here, Mum. Goodness, I've worked in both the hospital and street clinic. I've walked around. I've been in London. I've seen the worst side of life."

"But there's a difference. We have more support here to match the difficulties we encounter."

"Not always, Mum." Ethel remembered patients who had left the clinic clutching fevered children, heading for cold flats. "Anyway, from everything I've read, Canada is very inviting. You make it sound depressing."

"*Reality* is what I'm suggesting. And there's something else you should think about besides facilities and professions. Attitudes can be very different. I've read where women are encouraged to stay at home and look after their husband and family. We do that too, but it's more acceptable here for our class of women to work outside the home."

"What are you saying, Mum? That I won't be able to nurse?"

Mum cleared her throat. "I'm not saying that, dear. But I do know that attitudes will be different. A woman might be expected to encourage her man and work alongside him; certainly in the country I would think that'd be the case. You have to remember, here in England we can't even vote or own property. And if that isn't enough, the government can't quite decide if we've got a mind. I hear they're going to vote if we're even persons, and that probably won't happen for decades."

"How could that be? Women are women wherever they are. A country can't dictate a person's worth or declare how a woman should live her life. Surely, women's needs are the same, regardless of where they live." Uncertainty crept through Ethel like a cold chill. She wished she'd thought about these things before, yet still hoping she could share her opinions openly in Canada. Contradictory understandings about issues affecting the home and community had never limited her voice, and she didn't want it to begin now.

"I have my nursing certificate, and I've worked alongside the best." Ethel centred a wooden bowl on the table, running her fingers over her father's carefully hand-hewn edges. "I remember hearing about England's Midwives Act of 1902, long before I thought it possible for me to train as a practical nurse. Surely there'll be something in Canada by now."

"I'm only telling you what I read about the West, right in their posters and advertisements." Mum tapped a flyer lying on the table. "Nursing has definitely taken great strides, but you have to remember it's only been the last few years that nurses could care for men, look after them, and that's thanks to Miss Nightingale."

"I know, Mum, but it's different now. This is the 1900s." Ethel sighed. Her immediate concerns were for Elsie and Tom, but she also wanted to nurse in the future. All through the planning with Tom, the conversations at the clinic and with the doctor, Ethel had never thought once that attitudes towards women might be different in Canada. In London, women had a voice, although not a terribly strong one. Still, they did speak out.

Several days later, Ethel set out to talk to the doctor again. She boarded the train to London, flopped onto a seat and rested her head against the back. The noise of the great iron beast filled her senses, and the clanging and banging echoed her confused feelings. Engine fumes saturated the air, leaving a putrid taste in her mouth, reminding her that some things in life aren't pleasant. She sighed and wondered about the advertisements for Canadian domestic servants. She'd worked in a big house caring for three children after grade school. No! She was a practical nurse. It was her calling.

Doctor Austin welcomed Ethel on her arrival to his office and invited her to sit. He promptly asked if she were there to talk further about Elsie.

"I am beginning to come to terms with your instruction, Doctor, although I think it will be the most difficult experience I will ever have in my entire life."

"I do not doubt that, Miss Kemp. I do hope it will not be for long."

Doctor Austin responded to Ethel's questions about Canadian employment and attitude by reminding her of Alberta's recently formed Canadian National Association of Trained Nurses, suggesting she find out about it and register with them.

She would have liked to obtain her British midwifery registration before leaving England, but that opportunity wouldn't happen for another year.

"Do you think the medical association will license midwives in Canada too?" Ethel asked.

Looking Ahead

The doctor responded, "Licensing is needed, as it regulates the practice and makes the midwives more accountable to a governing body beyond themselves." Straightening his tie, he appeared certain. "The other side of that argument is that it limits the freedom midwives have to help other women."

Ethel knew there were many women that shouldn't be attending births. Midwifery was such an old art—handed down from one generation to another.

"In the beginning," the doctor continued, "it was the most natural and expected service: women helping women. Over time, the church tried to take charge, and then the civil authorities."

"Midwives encourage women to labour more openly, don't you think? As their bodies demand, you know. And many doctors, like yourself, have learned the value in that," Ethel said without waiting for the doctor to respond. Shifting her position and raising her eyebrows, she continued rather boldly, "In the future, midwifery will be a natural part of nursing—without additional training. They should go hand in hand. It's just instinct. Even in the time of Moses, God commended the midwives. I think this age or place is no different—just the laws and some countries. One day, nurses will be midwives with pride, and again, God—and country—will commend them. It's just a matter of time. I hope I'm around to see it."

Doctor Austin laughed, appearing to enjoy her forthrightness and wit. "I hope so too. You just keep that grit and vigour. It'll fit in fine over there. They need your kind in the cities and on the prairies. You'll see." He lifted his hand to shake hers. "I believe in you, Miss Kemp. You'll probably change some attitudes. You know, women have been doing that a lot lately, both here and in Canada. When you get over there, listen hard. Keep in line with what's expected of you, but look for opportunities to speak your mind. You'll be fine."

Later in the afternoon, the train moved out of the station, hissing and chugging, giving Ethel an exceptionally rough ride home. She settled into the corner of the seat, hoping to brace her body for the jolting. Women came to her mind who had fostered her independent spirit, ones who had answered needs in communities by founding private nursing homes and opening clinics. She wanted that kind of opportunity too. She wanted to help other women labour, raise their children, make decisions and provide good homes. Someday she'd have her own clinic in Canada. When she arrived, she'd see about her nursing status as soon as possible, find other work in the meantime and take one day at a time.

For now, Ethel vowed to spend extra time with Elsie and explain that the doctor wanted her to stay with her grandparents until she was completely healed. This would be a special time. Today she would tell Elsie that her mummy must go to Canada to find her pa, and together they would prepare a home where she would come as soon as possible. Ethel would promise her lots of letters and clippings of pictures from the local newspaper. In all of this, Ethel prayed that God would bridge the space between them and keep them bonded.

Her shoulders relaxed, and she felt more peaceful—at least about some things. Pleasant scenes of gardens and cottages sped quickly by, and soon the gliding of the train along the tracks eased her into a restful sleep.

Ethel and Mum planned the farewell meal; they organized games and a few gifts for the family gathering. After checking to be sure the loo, attached to the back of the house, had fresh tissue paper, Ethel watched Mum walk past her geraniums and climbing rosebushes, tilting her head, obviously enjoying their familiar fragrance. Pa had tidied the garden and set out a few chairs in case anyone wanted to sit there. Everything was prepared.

The small house on Goat Lane filled to overflowing onto the front step. The sun warmed the air after a fresh rain, giving a comfortable temperature for the children to run in and out. Mum moved to and from the scullery, bringing food to the main living room to place on the big table. All nine of Ethel's siblings, from five years of age to mid twenties, bantered back and forth, making entertaining conversation, finishing each other's statements and sometimes overlapping their voices—chaos, but so like home at the best of times.

A couple of Ethel's sisters had asked to speak on behalf of the rest of the family, promising lots of laughter and tears to fill the afternoon. Ethel rehearsed the words she'd say, but she couldn't even practice them without crying. Squaring her shoulders, acknowledging that the task ahead would be difficult, she took a deep breath.

"You'll be sure to write to us, Etty," Ethel's sister Florence insisted. "I'm soon going into service, but I'll get home to read your letters."

"I will," Ethel said. "I'll write to all of you, and you can pass the letters around. And somebody please write and tell me all about Mabel's wedding. She'll be too busy being married to write…" The family's laughter rose above the rest of the words.

Mabel stood and bowed gracefully. "And that big day will happen on October 25th at the register office. I wish you were going to be here, Ethel, but

Looking Ahead

I'll excuse you, only because I'll have my namesake here to carry the rings." Everybody looked over at Elsie, who smiled back. "Remember," Mabel continued, "my full name is Mabel *Elsie* Kemp. But folks, we're here because of Ethel, so let's ask her for a word."

All eyes turned towards Ethel. She took a deep breath and looked toward Mum and Pa and then across her siblings' faces one at a time as if savouring each expression. Moving closer to Elsie, she said, "The time has come for me to leave for Canada, and Elsie will stay here with Mum and the rest of you." She wiped her tears away with the back of her hand. "I can hardly bear it."

"I cannot imagine how heartbroken you are, having to go alone," Mabel said, reaching out to take Ethel's hand.

"Maybe when she can travel, one of us'll get to take her over," Ethel's 17-year-old brother, Ernie, added.

"We'll hold you to that, son," Pa said. "Even though it makes me sad at the thought, I know there will be great opportunity for you in Canada." He moved over and made room for the little girls to stand in front of him. "In the meantime, Horace'll take good care of you, Etty. He'll put you on the ship and give you a fine send-off."

Ethel smiled over at Horace, who looked back with a comical grin, and said, "And for you, dear brother, I'll be eternally grateful. I didn't relish walking those Liverpool docks on my own." She looked back at Pa and then to Ernie adding, "Nothing will please me more than getting Elsie over and seeing whoever brings her." Ethel put her hand in her pocket and pulled out a handkerchief. "And, you've got a bed however long you want to stay." She held her breath to keep from sobbing. Silence filled the room.

"We love you, big sister," Edith said. "We're going to miss you,"

"Come on now, everybody. I know you've all shed a river of tears, and there's time for more later," Mum said, "but right now, the food's hot and waiting. Let's make this a feast to remember." Turning, she continued, "Pa, please ask God to bless the food, Ethel, her journey…and to sanction all these tears."

Silence fell around them as if hemming them in. The children moved in beside their parents, and some of them held hands. Ethel felt the preciousness of the moment as she gripped her mother's arm with one hand and laid the other on top of Elsie's soft curls. Pa cleared his voice and began to speak softly. Ethel could hear the love he had for his family woven through each word. The hum of voices in the final amen brought closure to more than the prayer.

The next morning Ethel looked across the breakfast table at Elsie turning her spoon around and around in her porridge. How discerning this child was—perhaps not capable of putting her feelings into words but showing them in her actions. Life over the last month had left Ethel feeling as if she too were turning in circles from one emotion to another.

She fixed her eyes on Elsie's face and thought how people always remarked on their likeness. She wasn't surprised at their comments, because those same people had said for years that Ethel was a mirror image of *her* mother. She knew it to be true as she looked over at Mum and smiled. Those beautiful facial features framed by her lovely soft dark hair resembled Ethel's own countenance in many ways. Three generations, and so much alike.

There was a lot to say in these last few minutes before Ethel would leave for the train station, yet the silence allowed these deep thoughts to penetrate her mind. Looking at Elsie and then back to her mother, Ethel knew she'd see Elsie again, but the awful truth surfaced that leaving Mum was different. Saying goodbye to Pa earlier when he went to work had almost crushed Ethel, and now the same turmoil between what she wanted and what she must do divided her loyalties again. She doubted if she'd ever get back to England in her parents' lifetime, and she knew they wouldn't make the trip to Canada.

Breaking the silence, Ethel looked for words to move her past this moment of despair. "I'll write letters to you both while I'm still on the boat and post them as soon as I land."

"That will be lovely, dear," Mum said. "The whole family will gather to read them." Tears ran down her reddened cheeks.

"And you, luv." Ethel reached over to Elsie, lifted her from the chair and drew her close. "Come and sit on your mummy's knee." She turned her face towards her own. "What shall I send you when I get to Canada?"

"Can you send me kisses?" Elsie asked.

"Do you mean those chocolate candy kisses?" Ethel laughed. "For your sweet tooth?"

"Yes, 'n some of these," Elsie said quietly and placed her fingers on Ethel's lips.

Ethel pushed her face into Elsie's hair, more to hide her own tears than to whisper. "I'll find a way to send you something special, sweetheart, with Mummy's kisses all over it."

She straightened and glanced at the kitchen clock ticking away precious minutes and then looked at Mum. Ethel's bottom lip trembled. She wanted to bawl—just rest her head on the table as if she were alone and cry until there were no tears left.

Just then, Horace came into the living room, twirling his peak cap between his fingers. "We've got a bit of a trip ahead of us, Etty. Are you ready to go?"

"I think I am," Ethel replied. "As ready as I'll ever be."

"Ethel," Mum said, "you know I support you in this decision, and I'll follow you all the way to the dock in my heart, through my thoughts and in my prayers. When I close my eyes over the long hours to come, I'll see you with your shoulders straight and holding your head high." She paused to brush a tear from her cheek and said softly, "We'll all be with you in spirit, lass. Know that you are loved, and no miles, no distance, absolutely nothing can change that."

"Oh Mum." Ethel sighed. "What will I do without you and your words of wisdom? Is there anything that will make this easier?"

"Nothing is going to help, my dear, unless you decide to bring your luggage back from the train station, unpack your clothes and stay put here in Enfield." Mum attempted a weak smile while wiping her eyes. "And that's not going to happen. So we just have to get through this."

Mum stood and linked her fingers around Horace's elbow. "In the meantime, Horace will look after you until you board the ship." She stood on her tiptoes and kissed him on the cheek. "That'll settle my mind, some."

Elsie squirmed in Ethel's arms, and Ethel tightened her grip as she listened to Mum.

"Once you get on the boat, you'll start thinking of the immediate and of Tom, you'll see. I've heard others say the same thing. It's just getting you to the dock and onto that ship." She bent over and placed her hand on Ethel's face. "And keep the faith, lass. Remember the Scripture you were raised with."

"I will, Mum. I'll always remember that."

Reluctantly, Ethel let Elsie down. She stood and leaned over to embrace Mum, resting her head on Mum's shoulder as she did when a child. She knew to which Scripture Mum alluded. There'd be no problem loving her neighbour as herself, but she didn't know if she could love God today with all her heart and soul and might. She'd prayed so much about Elsie's health, and it had only worsened. Indeed, she would have to talk to God more about that.

Ethel turned to Elsie, knelt and lowered her face into her little girl's neck. She recalled the long and difficult struggle of giving birth and then holding Elsie's sweet stirring body, bundled up in soft flannelette.

She drank in the sight and familiar scent of her little girl and looked into her pleading eyes. Cupping Elsie's face in her hand, she kissed her forehead with a long, lingering touch. "Goodbye, my dearest, for now."

Nurse Rankin's words about good things coming from labour pains flashed through her mind. What could possibly come out of this pain except more of the same?

With that, Ethel kissed Elsie again and turned her toward Mum. She picked up her purse and said, "Let's go, Horace. You and me, we'll make good use of our extra time together. You can tell Mum all about it when you return." She grabbed her satchel by the handles, pushed the kitchen door with her free hand and walked out into the sunshine. Glancing back for one more look, Ethel saw Mum in the doorway holding Elsie, who was eagerly waving a white handkerchief. "I'm wavin' it like they do on boats, Mummy."

"Thank you, sweetheart," Ethel said as she swallowed her tears. "I'll think of this when I board the ship."

chapter four

Grief in Goodbye

The wheels clattered over the uneven railway sleepers on the tracks, changing to the screeching sound of iron on iron—rubbing, dragging, seizing. Ethel and Horace chatted comfortably while bumping along in the passenger coach as it rumbled and swayed on the tracks towards Liverpool. They'd caught the train at Enfield Town Station without problem, and now the occasional mournful call of the train whistle seemed to widen the distance between Ethel and her family. Tiny droplets of rain slid down the window, disappearing out of sight. Ethel watched while thinking that nothing stays forever. During this daylong trip to Liverpool, she'd have a lot of thinking time.

The train slipped through back gardens, towns and industrial settings. She took some sandwiches Mum had made from her satchel and opened two jars of fresh water and handed one to Horace. They lunched while looking at the daily newspaper and commenting on the scenery. After brushing away the crumbs and putting the soiled paper into the waste, Ethel rested her head back on the seat as her muddled thoughts became one with the rumbling sound of the train. Laughing and talking about their childhood filled the hours, and Ethel cherished each one as a gift with Horace.

Wrapping her arms around her body, as if to nurture and strengthen a less than confident spirit to uphold her during the time ahead, she felt the reduced speed of the train. The scenery had changed, and they had entered the heavily populated centre of Liverpool: buildings, smokestacks and multiple train tracks.

"Are we here?" Ethel asked.

"Almost," Horace replied. "Thanks for this extra time, sis. It's been good."

"Yes, it has been." Ethel began to gather her bags together. "It's so peaceful just riding along with you."

"Not like when we were kids and you were always teasing me." Horace laughed a hearty chuckle.

"Ah, it wasn't that bad." Ethel looked at him, soaking in her brother's jovial facial features. It was so kind of him to make this trip over to Liverpool with her. But then, that was who he was: fun-loving and kindhearted. How she appreciated him.

As the train slowly moved into the station, steam filled the window view. Ethel began to organize her things. "The station porter will help us to get off and pick up the luggage," Horace said gently to Ethel. "We'll ask where the closest respectable boarding house is and get ourselves a hot meal. Would you like that?"

"I would indeed," Ethel replied. "I feel a little like leftover laundry, crumpled and wrinkled."

"You look just fine to me, sis," Horace said and winked at her.

They made their way off the train and walked into the station, looking for someone who could give them directions. Indeed, a good meal and a place to sleep were welcome. Ethel knew tomorrow would be filled with a greater challenge. Would she be ready for it?

Ethel's buttoned boots, newly repaired and perfectly polished, poked out from under the hemline of her lightweight tweed skirt. Her hair was parted enough to the side to allow a few curls to fall around her face under her hat; a delicately ingrained ivory comb firmly held the rest in place. She laid a wool wrap over the sleeve of her favourite high-buttoned cotton blouse, ready for the brisk harbour wind. Pa had told her that even in July she needed to prepare for the dampness in the air.

After she and Horace had followed the directions from the boarding house to the dock, Ethel raised her hand to shade her eyes from the July sunrays that filtered through the grey clouds and danced across the open water. As they walked along the stone pavement, she noticed the hectic pace of the dock.

"Are you surprised how busy these docks are?" Horace asked.

"Not really," Ethel responded. "I've read of the enormous basins and miles of railroads. Liverpool docks are active and noisy."

"This would be an exciting place to be any other day, Etty, but today, it's a lot different for you, eh?" Horace said.

"You're right about that," Ethel said realizing they were like a gate slowly closing to separate her from loved ones on this side of the Atlantic Ocean.

Grief in Goodbye

Massive crates waiting on the dock to be loaded sheltered them from the wind as they walked toward the huge passageway, while the dockworkers yelled orders. The grand ocean liner SS *Lake Manitoba* gently pushed the water against the wet dockside, leaving ripples in its black reflection. Securely anchored in the murky water and tied to the dock through large steel rings, it stood ready. Several tugboats hung back, prepared to pull it out into the mouth of the River Mersey for its ten-day passage.

The smell of fumes mixed with fish, wet wood and rope made Ethel resist swallowing the phlegm in her throat. It left a foul taste in her mouth. She looked up at this enormous ship, knowing that in minutes she'd go on-board and change her life forever. Although physically prepared to join the other passengers on the ship, throbs of isolation and helplessness suddenly gripped her like a vise.

She didn't think she had any tears left, but when she turned to Horace, who was usually full of fun and tricks, she saw tears in his eyes. "You have a good heart, brother of mine. I'll always be grateful to you for bringing me here and seeing me safely onto the ship." After hugging him, she stepped onto the gangplank and walked towards the upper deck.

chapter five

Watching Life Change

"You'd better make your way down to your quarters, ma'am."

Ethel turned to face a cloud of mint-scented tobacco. A man with a wool peak cap set on a ridge of fuzzy short hair looked kindly at her. "It can get pushy down there. Some people get pretty nasty about protecting their space. Just claim yours and stay quiet. Hang on to it and you'll be fine."

He was right. Steerage, or third class as it was now called, would be a challenge, but it would have to wait. Ethel couldn't bring herself to move. The wind played along the deck and wrapped around her skirt. At times, familiar strains of "Guide Me O Thou Great Jehovah" filtered from the large crowd singing from the dock and brought her a sense of well-being, even in the midst of grief. The ship jolted, and although she couldn't feel any actual movement, the shudder told her the vessel had been set in motion.

A feeling of panic pulsed throughout her body. Looking into what seemed to be bottomless water, she thought of her life. In her frantic moments of facing the possibility of never seeing Elsie again, she identified with its dark, cold, unknown depth. Like a magnet drawn to steel, she dropped her gaze down into the dark water that reflected her worst fears. The time between now and seeing Elsie again would be the most difficult to live, and perhaps the most complicated to explain.

The majestic steamship soon began to slice through the water, unhurriedly at first and then changing to a smooth flowing motion as it followed the little tugboats. The floating sensation slowly carried Ethel away from the waving white handkerchiefs, balloons and signs. She clung tightly with one hand to the wooden rail that separated her from the deep and formidable waters of the harbour; the other hand clutched her waist, as if needing to feel the warmth of her body.

Moaning sounds from the ship's foghorn joined with the chatter of voices interrupted her thoughts, and the moist channel air reached deep into her lungs. She turned her face toward the fog that looked like a protective quilt stretched across a clothesline, sealing off this part of her life. Tears burned, continually flooding her eyes and obscuring her sight as she strained to capture the fading view of the dock. She angrily wiped them away so they wouldn't blur her vision—she wanted to catch every movement on the shore. Just knowing Horace was standing there in that massive crowd watching gave her a sense of peace, filling her with love. And even though she could no longer see their faces, the memory of Elsie sitting in her grandmother's arm at their cottage door, waving a white handkerchief in unbroken rhythm, pretending to be standing on the dock, remained indelible in her mind.

In spite of the wind, passengers on the great deck shoved and pushed against her for a space to see the fast-fading Liverpool port diminish in size.

"Nothing more to see now, folks. Might as well go down," one of the deckhands said.

"I might never see this again," Ethel said. "I guess I'm trying to savour some memories."

"I'll tell you what's going to happen," he said, pointing to the shoreline. "Those tall towers and buildings over there, they're gonna fade from sight; the windows of those warehouses will dull until you can't even see them; and all those layers of shaded roofs are just gonna look like miniature boxes. I've seen this change many times. Even those marshlands that border the River Mersey will turn grey when it widens out to join the open sea. Believe me, nothing special to see. Might as well go in. Gonna get cold when we get out a bit. Better git yourself on down." The man nattered as if he'd said it a thousand times.

Gulls called as they dipped up and down from the waves, adding their squawking to Ethel's silent cry. The imposing steamer, now on its own power, glided through the shimmering waters and continued to move away from her homeland.

Ethel pulled her cloak tightly around her shoulders, shielding herself from the damp air. Thankful the porters had already taken her trunks below, she lifted two small satchels and made her way towards the big double doors, along with the remaining passengers. Having stayed up on the deck a little too long, she pushed and shoved her way down the stairs, determined to secure accommodations. It was not unheard of for a woman to travel alone, but Ethel, even with her confidence, was uncomfortable.

Watching Life Change

Proud that she'd been careful with her funds, she'd put aside six pounds to cover her passage, the five-dollar landing fee after she landed in Quebec and sufficient fare for her trip west. She knew her fare had a British Bonus Allowance applied to the total amount, but she couldn't benefit from it until she was settled as an immigrant. However, waves of positive memories filled her as she remembered the refund she'd been able to add to her savings when she changed her accommodation down from second class. Although she would have rather had it used for its initial purpose, she added the reimbursement from the cancellation of Elsie's ticket to her total funds. It'd be a while before she'd find work in Edmonton, and she would be careful with her finances.

Stepping carefully along the passageway, she followed people through a long common room. Children whined, and Ethel watched them grip their parents' hands. Old people shuffled and pushed, some dropping their bags while others dragged theirs. She could surely help some of these people later.

Ethel saw a compartment with a small storage area and moved toward the bunk ahead of her. Looking around, she decided it wasn't so bad, since the railing was high enough to give some privacy. She sat on the bottom bunk and after a few minutes opened her satchel and began to arrange her personal things in neat piles.

Her journal lay begging for attention. Maybe she'd write some things down that she could copy into a letter at another time.

> The mattress isn't much thicker than Mum's back door mat. I guess a roll of what seems like a sheaf of cotton is my pillow. And a blanket not unlike what the neighbour would use on his horse is folded across the bottom of the cot. I think about fleas and lice and then I remember the ship's new rules of disinfecting all cloth goods.
>
> I'm pleased with my space. Everything is quite contained: wooden bunk bed, a little bit of floor space with room for personals, and a small aisle leads out to an area where passengers can cook food and heat water. There's a toilet and basin in an adjoining alcove quite close to my area; even now, it seems crowded with people.
>
> I can see a bigger open area, I guess for small groups for visiting, playing music and cards. And I suppose for teaching purposes if children want to do their sums. There's a good supply of candles on a shelf, should the oil lamps burn dry. This space is not terribly pleasant, but liveable.

> I read a sign that there is salted meat, water, bread, oatmeal and ship's biscuits included with the fare. I suspect as time goes on, supplies will become meagre and stale. I remember hearing horror stories about steerage accommodation in the big steamers. Organization and security in these smaller quarters will be important. The stagnant air causes me some concern, but I'll go up on deck to get relief.
>
> One of Tom's letters comes to my mind. He said, "Doctor Austin told me that my asthma was controllable. 'Good clean air and a different environment will make you a new man.'" But Tom had mentioned that it was hard to find fresh air in steerage.

Ethel closed her journal for the time being, looked at her hair combs and creams and sorted some small pictures along with a few keepsakes. She opened her satchel again, checked some clothes and folded them. While unwrapping a small nativity scene, hand carved by her father, special memories came back to her. Tucking her mother's geranium slips deeper into their moist paper and soil, she hoped they'd survive the journey.

Handling several pieces of jewellery that Mum had given her, Ethel was relieved she'd packed them. Sisters Mabel, Edith and Florence had appreciated the little things she'd given them, and of course, Mum had cried when Ethel left her some needlework.

Ethel lifted a picture of Elsie wearing a long white christening dress, a gift from Tom's parents, her shawl and bonnet hand-knit by Mum. She brushed away tears that slipped down her cheeks. There'd be so much she'd miss in Elsie's early years, but her christening day in St. Andrew's, Church of England would be a cherished remembrance. She was happy she'd posted Tom a copy at the time.

Ethel re-opened her journal and smiled as she thought about her mother's last embrace:

> When Mum put her arms around me, it caused me to remember the happy, simple and honest home of my childhood. Pa, bless his heart, was a hard worker, changing jobs whenever he had to for a continuous paycheque. His attitude and polite nature helped us to thrive through difficult times. He provided the best he could and taught all of us to work hard to accomplish goals and achieve in life. He and Mum raised a big family in a loving and frugal environment: plain, but with

everything we needed, including lots of encouragement and love. They grieved Will's death together and always included us in their sorrow so we could share our sadness.

Later as Ethel settled on her cot, her gentle rhythm of breathing comforted her. She could feel the working motion of the ship, its pressured pace in obedience to engines somewhere beyond the walls. She felt strangely comforted by the regularity and movement. The consistent creaking of the ship's hull echoed as it took the brunt of ocean waves. Rolling over, Ethel began to think of herself as in a large cradle rocking back and forth.

Sobs, giggles, snores and muffled sounds resonated through the larger space as people settled and filled the darkness of the first night. She ran her tongue across her top lip, tasting her salty tears, and thought of the vast ocean of salt water: her grief compared.

Ethel breathed deeply. "Goodnight, Elsie, my precious. Keep well. Stay safe. God be with you until we meet again." When she woke up, she'd be miles closer to Canada. Yes, that's the way it had to be—thoughts about Canada.

chapter six

Settling In

Ethel awakened to shadows. Elsie's face came to her memory, and Ethel's eyes watered. The emotional darkness that had kept her company over the last few weeks was nearby, but she managed to set it aside to think about the day ahead. Stretching, she looked around the space.

People were already moving, groaning and shifting trunks across the wooden floors as Ethel swung her legs over the side of the bunk, stood and straightened her clothes. She went into the common room and washed her hands, glad the tap was working. Applying some hand lotion to sooth the stinging from the salt water, she looked up and smiled at those standing around her. Back in her space, she made up her bed and laid her food portions out for breakfast. She peeled a piece of fruit, put it on a thick piece of bread and then ate it. Breakfast was to be in the common room tomorrow, where, the word was, they'd have ship's porridge.

Ethel had escaped the immediate problem of seasickness that was sweeping across people like a buffeting wave. At least it would force their minds off their homesickness. She listened to them moaning and vomiting and wondered if there would be adequate water to clean after them.

During the first day at sea, Ethel heard there were 737 passengers on board the SS *Lake Manitoba*. It was like having a floating town. She couldn't imagine that many people in one boat and thought of the germs that could spread in such a situation. Although terribly grateful the cargo of cattle was at the opposite end of the ship, she pictured the eager Canadian farmers waiting at the stable markets on docking.

After another day, people began to recover from seasickness; some moved around, some complained bitterly, some sulked and kept to themselves, while others tried to make light conversation.

A couple of the men brought out their fiddles and played several tunes. Some of the women laid out board games in the common room. Children had a variety of toys to keep them busy. For the most part, activities made the time past quickly.

Early on the fourth day, Ethel moved around more to see how others were faring. Just as she sat down at one of the tables in the common room, two people began to talk loudly.

"There's poison in the air, I tell ya," one man said slowly. "I can feel it."

"Naw, you've been reading too much propaganda," his female companion said.

"The newspapers say there's some smelly politics goin' on. I read about it before we left 'ome. That'll mean money problems, you'll see. Trouble marks the British air. Aye! I heard them speeches. Some of the boys down at the pub 'ave been talkin' 'bout war. Does 'e think this could be a hint of somethin'?" He raised his voice. "They'd better git out 'n leave them posh chairs 'n talk to us ordinary people. We'll tell 'em a thing or two."

Ethel thought about the man's comment and asked a woman next to her, "There hasn't been a lot of talk about war, has there?"

"Not really. Political power shifts, poverty, industrial problems and rising financial concerns are all current issues, but I guess war is always a question when it comes to who wants the power."

"I don't like the talk of war. Do you think it'll ever happen?" Ethel asked. The thought of being separated from Elsie in a time of peace was bad enough. But war? She couldn't imagine it.

"That's fear talking," the woman said. "Won't be for a while."

Tucking that thought away in her mind, Ethel decided to go for a walk. Children played on the floor together, obviously not influenced by adult fears. They were completely absorbed in their game of jacks. Some little girls ran and played around their mum's knees. How blessed they were to travel together.

Sleeping and talking seemed to fill Ethel's days. Several families in the surrounding sections had left children for educational, health or financial reasons, but even hearing that didn't ease Ethel's anguish. Memories of relationships in England saddened her, and she often changed the subject.

Ethel walked on the steerage deck and the air blew fresh against her skin. The sunset boasted wide strips of grey across the okra sky, presenting a kaleidoscope

Settling In

of colour. The sky looked like a grand canopy. Thinking about her colleagues at the hospital and the various patients she'd grown fond of during her employment gave her a burst of encouragement. She hadn't had many friends, just her family and fellow nurses. Perhaps it will be the same in Canada—but she hoped for friends. She breathed deeply and pulled her scarf around her neck as she turned back toward her sleeping quarters.

Ethel lay on the bunk bed that night feeling a new comfort within the ship's walls as its continuous movement rocked her. She thought about the prospect of nursing in Edmonton and remembered when that idea had intimidated her. On the crossing she'd been able to comfort several people, assist with a birth and share some of her home remedies. This had renewed her confidence about nursing in difficult situations. She'd met people who impressed her, disgusted her and blessed her, but she was glad to help all of them.

The weather for the first part of the trip had offered fair skies, but not so for the latter.

"The winds have picked up out of the south. We're fighting them at seventy miles an hour," a loud voice echoed through her quarters in the early morning.

The vessel rolled and pitched. Word travelled fast that the ship was taking on water over the forward deck, and water was crashing against the portholes. People passed news around that men had secured the decks with ropes and chains to reduce stress and keep control as they worked to maintain their course.

"Remember the man talking about ships having to catch waves at an angle during ocean storms? That's got to take a bit of know-how," Ethel said to the woman beside her at breakfast.

"I know. I heard them too. One even talked about the risk of capsizing if the captain heads straight into the waves. Said he was afraid of breaking up the ship. We'll know it if he chooses to take the waves broadside."

"How in the world can they manoeuvre a ship this size to do that?"

"I guess that's why we're passengers," a man replied, "and those men up there are doing their job. Now, don't worry. We'll be fine."

Murmuring a prayer for the captain and those fighting the elements on deck, Ethel decided to stay at the table awhile and visit with the women.

For forty hours, the wind howled and the waves crashed. Ethel stayed in her quarters for the most part. Only quiet prayer had the power to silence her anxiety as wailing filled the cavity of the ship.

Reaching deep into the pockets of her skirt, she retrieved the note Pa had

A Rare Find

given her. She knew it would offer encouragement. "When the sea gets rough, Ethel, remember the promises of God: 'For this shall every one that is godly pray unto thee in a time when thou mayest be found: surely in the floods of great waters they shall not come nigh unto him' (Psalm 32:6)."

This was comforting during the storm. Stories of other ships that had taken their passengers to ocean graves did not escape her thoughts, but she trusted that today would be different.

When the storm was over, Ethel felt bonded to the people as in a family, hope being the common tie. The captain announced they were a little off their course but would be able to make up the time. During that day, Ethel moved around the area to see how other people had coped with their fears during the wretched storm.

Several days passed before a steward came to the common room, announced that they had entered the St. Lawrence river and that land lay ahead. Ethel could see the excitement heighten among some of the passengers, while fear developed into tears for others, especially those who had been sick and feared a health inspection.

She went up on deck and joined the chorus of people hollering, "Land! Land! We see land!" Ethel strained her eyes but couldn't see anything. She looked over the water, anticipating what lay ahead. And then, squinting, she saw the horizon, and within the hour it filled with shapes like little boxes. What a glorious sight! The ship seemed to be moving faster, although she doubted that to be the case.

"Do you see what I see?" Ethel laughed as she stood on the deck with some folks. "It's Canada, isn't it?"

"It is," a woman said, "and none too soon, I'd say. I can hardly wait to step onto Canadian soil."

Over the next few hours, Grosse Isle shore came into full view, and Ethel saw buildings of different shapes, sizes and colours. Various shades of turquoise and deep blues gave the ocean a serene appearance. Ethel smiled, remembering the storm they had come through. She lifted her head to face the fresh breeze; Canadian air, warm and comforting, blew against her face. The ship passed small islands and buildings along the shoreline that carved out the horizon. Sea spray deposited a refreshing cover of moisture over Ethel as she watched.

Seagulls soared up and down, skimming the water and resting on the ripples, waiting to lift up again. The water moved gracefully, obedient to the wind, and a smooth surface of distinct colour beckoned the ship onward. As beautiful as the water appeared, it was taking her closer to her own fears on shore—the dreaded health inspection station. Ethel thought this was a little like life; experiences that you have to go through are often a barrier to where you want to go.

"Canada, it's the true north strong and free," Ethel said to no one in particular.

"From what I've read about this place, we'll need all the strength we can muster to begin that gruelling process ahead," a man growled from behind her.

Ethel agreed silently, and then, remembering her morning prayers, she said a word of thanks before pulling her scarf tightly around her head.

chapter seven

One Step After Another

The captain asked the passengers to go back down to their compartments until it was their turn to go ashore. Fear soon robbed Ethel of her excitement of seeing land as she remembered stories of inspectors turning people back, dividing families, freeing some to go on to their destination and forcing others to return to their homeland.

When the time came to board the ferry, she ascended the stairs from her compartment, jostled along by other passengers. She welcomed the warm sun on her face as she looked at the barren terrain spread before her.

Ethel had read about this entrance to Canada, and she knew she wasn't far from landing. The grand ship anchored in the river, away from the shore but close enough for Ethel to make out the outline of buildings on the island. A ridge of trees made the place look peaceful; maybe that was because of all those graves she'd heard about. The inspection station windows reflected the morning sun. Mum would like that shine if she were here.

"Come on, move. Shove your way in," a deckhand shouted. "There ain't any more boats—this 'ere's the last one. If you want to git to the inspection station, you better squeeze in."

Ethel wiggled into position, noticing that some people shook with fear while a few giggled from embarrassment or apologized for cramping the space more with their presence. Excited children with high-pitched voices called back and forth to one another, obviously forgetting about previous gruelling days and now only thinking about the new land.

"This ferry smells of rotten wood and fish," Ethel grumbled, "and it looks so old, it's about to sink."

The excitement of a new country, a new opportunity, now seemed secondary to her. Getting through the inspection was foremost in her mind.

Tension cut through her thoughts. She sat, head down, thinking, feeling tired…like a refugee…a second-class citizen. What must she look like after all those days in the belly of the ship?

When the boat docked, Ethel stepped out and onto the gangplank that led up to the inspection building. Men in long grey cotton coats holding paper pads stood along the railings. She knew they'd be watching for any signs of visible weakness: a limp, a cough, a person leaning on another, anyone crying or being overtly quiet would draw their attention. They watched. They noted.

She missed Tom's positive attitude and sense of humour at a time like this. She felt so alone. Women attendants shouted orders. Large printed signs gave direction: "To the showers." "Undress. Put clothes in bags." "Remember your number." "Keep moving." A harsh voice herded the female passengers into rooms like animals, then ordered them to drop their clothes, stuff them in the net bags and move on. A cold spray hit Ethel's back. Frowning, she turned to see where it had come from and faced the full impact of disinfectant.

"Can't you tell a body when you're going to do that?" she asked.

"Everybody has the same chance. Read the signs. Listen to the orders. Move on. Now!"

The line seemed to get longer. The women and girls walked with their heads lowered, trying to be modest.

"What do they do with our clothes?" a woman asked Ethel as she walked up beside her.

"They're going to get a good steaming. Apparently it doesn't take long," Ethel replied.

The big doors opened into the shower room. Showering was obviously a first experience for many of the women, as they appeared confused. The water coming out of the nozzle seemed to scare them, and they sidestepped the spray.

"Get under it! Under it, I said!" a woman attendant hollered. "Wash!"

Ethel saw the showers as a privilege as well as a necessity. She could hardly wait her turn, and when she stepped into the shower and felt the water flush over her, she closed her eyes and didn't want it to stop. The smell of the water filled her senses, and she hoped it would wash away her fears and fatigue as well as any lingering soil.

Too quickly, Ethel finished, and an attendant told her to dress. She pushed along a corridor with other women and children, some stumbling on their shoelaces as they walked out into the sunshine. Feeling refreshed, even if somewhat humiliated, Ethel left the shower house with a new vitality.

She recognized some of the people with whom she'd shared steerage and thought they looked somewhat relieved to have travelled this far. The inspection officers hollered directions and began to push the people into what looked like a holding pen for animals at the town market.

A man touched her shoulder and spoke through a megaphone. "Move on. Follow the arrows. One at a time, or a family—take your choice. Keep moving. Stay in your lines."

This steady lingo of words and orders continually rang in Ethel's ears. Signs on the wall directed her toward the examination areas where doctors waited. One of them ushered Ethel into a small cubicle, where several stainless steel instruments lay on an examining table. Her medical eye surveyed the contents of the room, trying to determine just what they did with people.

"Welcome to Canada," the officer said stiffly, reminding her of the lifeless voices in the hallways. "How was your trip?"

"It was long, but I was quite comfortable," Ethel answered.

"Did you have any problems in the shower house? Get your clothes back all right?" he asked, this time in an exaggerated monotone voice.

"I got along fine," Ethel replied.

"This won't take long," the man said. "I want you to stand straight in front of me. Turn your head to the left, and then to the right. Now lift your arms up high over your head. Now bend down and point your fingertips to the floor. Don't bend your knees. That's enough."

The inspector wrote down his findings. That kind of stretching felt good on Ethel's tight muscles. The man asked Ethel to be seated. He reached over, abruptly pulled the skin down at the corners of both eyes and then promptly made a note in his binder. He asked a number of questions about digestion, sleep habits and past diseases. When looking at her skin, her fingernails and in her mouth didn't cause him obvious concern, he went back to make more notes.

"You heading for the west are you?" he continued as he flipped through the pages of her application without looking up.

"Yes, sir. Catching the morning train to Edmonton."

"You have relatives out there?" Except for his tone of voice, which sounded like the predictable rhythm of a train coming into a station, the man appeared genuinely interested in her welfare.

"I do," Ethel replied.

"Are you travelling alone?"

"Yes, sir." He raised his eyebrows. Ethel lifted her chin. *Well, let him think what he likes.*

"A man meeting you?"

"Yes, sir!"

"Do you have your landing fee?"

"Yes," Ethel responded in a clear, deep voice, grateful she'd organized her plans so well.

"You have no major health problem to report at this time?" the inspector asked, looking intently at Ethel.

"That's right," she answered.

The officer smiled. "Carry on then, ma'am."

"Thank you," Ethel said and sighed. She walked toward the door without looking back and set her fears aside. The examination was thorough, but it had not been as degrading as some rumours had suggested. Ethel's first impression of Canada satisfied her. She began to think of Quebec City, her gateway to Canada.

Sometime later, she travelled to the main docks by a different ferry and received her papers and directions at customs. She moved proudly into the noise of the harbour-front and walked up the wooden walkway, trying to dismiss a feeling that the earth was somehow moving beneath it.

She was in Canada and so thankful. Ethel looked around; horses, buggies, trunks and people filled the noisy entrance. It didn't look much different from home, and she guessed folks were generally the same wherever you went, except maybe for talking differently. That she'd noticed already.

Ethel appreciated the facilities available to the steerage passengers—a large building with adequate rooms, limited hot water and eating accommodations. This gave her time to prepare for further travel, so she gladly took advantage of Canadian hospitality.

The next day, Ethel sat stiffly as the seven-car train steamed, whistled, chugged up hills and raced down ravines. The countryside looked lush with the freshness of recent rain. Green hills, fertile pastures and flowing rivers criss-crossed the landscape. Ethel watched with great interest as they passed through little towns, some beckoning the train to stop and add more passengers or take on fresh water and freight. She took time to write in her journal and look at a magazine, as well as sleep.

After they crossed from Quebec to Ontario and eventually Manitoba, the prairies stretched out for miles beside her; Ethel could hardly take in their vastness.

"The land—I never thought it'd be like this!" Ethel exclaimed to the couple sitting across from her. "I've never seen such beautiful country; everything is so wide and high." She turned her face upward and looked through the windowpane. "And look at that big sky."

After their long train ride of many days, Ethel welcomed the conductor's words that they had arrived in Edmonton and said goodbye to her companions. Now to find Tom!

She picked up her satchel, held it tightly and then walked down the aisle towards the steps leading to the platform. Bending, she peered through the windows, searching the waiting crowd for Tom's face. So many people appeared like a sea moving, swaying and tipping. Everyone was waving and cheering, creating great excitement. How would she find him in this crowd of people? And would she know him? After all it'd been four years, and he'd been sick. *Oh, dear God, help me find my Tom.*

People pushed Ethel in their haste, and she clung tightly to the seat backs. When she stood on the top step of the iron stairs, she paused and raised her hand over her eyes to shade them from the bright sunshine. Fear surged through her mind as thoughts of Tom unable to come to the station consumed her. Maybe he was too sick. Maybe he didn't get her letter in time.

"Move along, ma'am," the attendant said. "There's a lot of people behind you that are wanting to get off the train."

"Yes, of course," Ethel said, "it's just that—"

"Ethel, over here!" a voice jangled through the excitement of the crowd.

At that moment, she saw a long arm waving frantically in the air. She raised her hand to her face as if in disbelief and then stretched it into the air to return the greeting. She stepped down onto the wooden platform and pushed her way towards Tom. And then his arms were around her back, his kisses covering her face, and she was lost in time.

Ethel placed her hands on his face and through her tears gasped, "After all this time, I see you again. There were times when I didn't believe we would ever have this moment."

He hugged her tightly. "I never doubted it for a minute, luv. Come on now; let's get out of the way so others can greet their visitors." He led Ethel over to the corner of the train station. "It is so good to see you." He held her at arm's length. "I love you so much." Pushing her hat back on her forehead, he said, "Did you have a good voyage, and what about the train ride? And Elsie, do you have a picture of her?" He hugged Ethel again and said, "I have so many questions."

"And I am glad to see you too, and oh, Tom, my love for you never varied even when I wondered if…" Swallowing, she appeared to gulp for air, trying to reply. She took a deep breath. "Yes, to answer your question of the ocean voyage and the train ride—they were both good. And yes, I have a picture of Elsie. She sends her love to you—getting to be a big girl, she is."

Ethel picked the deliberately placed picture from her bag. "There you go, Tom. I knew this would be among your first questions." She handed him a picture and watched as his eyes filled with tears. He looked tenderly at Elsie, moved his fingers across her face, and his tears fell on his shirtsleeve.

"She is so lovely, Ethel," he said. "I missed so much by coming over first, didn't I?"

"We did what we had to do at the time," Ethel said. "You remember the doctor's orders, difficult as they were for us to hear. He's still the same way—that's why I'm here without Elsie today." She sighed and looked up at Tom. "Now we can work together to make things right between us and the church…and in time, with Elsie."

"I've got a pretty good start on that," Tom said. "I board with my landlord, who owns my butcher shop. It's a nice area, and not far from the hospital if you get a job over there. In the meantime, his sister has a few flats for rent that will give you a roof over your head until we can work something else out."

"Are you over your disappointment yet—about Elsie not coming, I mean?"

"When I got your letter, I couldn't believe it," he said. "I'd looked forward to seeing her for so long." He cleared his throat as if to hide his emotion. "But her health must come first. As soon as we're established and she is well enough, we'll send for her. Having a nice place so handy to a hospital will ease Doctor Austin's mind." He hugged Ethel again, sweeping her off her feet, "In the meantime, I have you, and for that I am truly thankful."

"And the feeling is mutual," Ethel said, returning his embrace. "We have our life ahead of us together."

Tom turned back towards the train that sat puffing at the station. "And now, let's get your trunk and get on with this life."

PART II
1911

chapter eight

Firming Up Their New Life

"Isn't it just the prettiest place you've ever seen, Tom?" Ethel opened a door to a small veranda on the west side of the building. She could see this being a favourite place for them to sit.

"It is, indeed, luv," Tom replied. "It'll suit us just fine."

"Let's take it then," Ethel said, looking at the fine wooden doors and floorboards.

Tom gave their new landlord a month's rent. After looking for some time, they had finally found a pleasant flat in a clean house. The sun spread warmth across the room through two nice-sized windows. Sparkling clean countertops and brightly upholstered chairs gave the place a homey appearance. Having some furniture already placed helped Ethel decide without hesitation. She looked around the room and remembered Mum's kitchen back home. This felt so right.

After the landlord left, Ethel walked from room to room, touching the door frames and opening closet doors. He'd made a definite point of saying that closets were often a scarcity in rented portions of larger homes, but this particular one had two of them. Moving to one of the windows, Ethel expanded her fingers across the sill, thinking about curtain material. She'd look after that as soon as possible.

She looked through the pane to the grounds below. "Mum'll rest easier knowing we're settled. I'll write her a letter after we move."

Sitting at their small kitchen table later in the week, Ethel penned a letter telling her mother the new address along with all the recent news, knowing she'd pass it on to Tom's folks.

August 1911

Dear Mum and everybody,

How are you? I hope you've been receiving my letters. It's been too long since I've written. I'm sorry for that. It's over a year since I came to Canada, and life is finally beginning to come together for us. I don't know why it has to be so difficult sometimes. It seemed we went two steps ahead and then one back. Since my last letter, we've made considerable changes, and we're both getting along well.

For the first time since I've left England, I feel a sense of security and comfort. I have a housekeeping job one day a week and I'm nursing at the local clinic for an additional two days each week. We have a lovely flat with a nice view, which is hard to get in the depth of the city. And you'll be glad to know, Mum, that we visited the priest at All Saint's Anglican Church—that's the same as the Church of England at home—and asked for God's blessing. Our two friends stood with us, and the priest performed a lovely wedding service. We've found a nice church fellowship right here on our street. I think we're really going to like it.

I hope that you're enjoying the summer months. They go too quickly, and soon the snow will be falling. My first winter in Canada was dreadful. You will remember from my past letters how ill-prepared I was for the season. However, now with the lovely warm months, I've forgotten the harsh winds of winter.

Tom is feeling a lot better than he was when I previously wrote. He has some new medicine from his doctor, and it seems to be helping his breathing. Although he tires easily, he is very careful not to overdo it.

I will write again soon. Please send me all the news. And say hello to the family. Give Mabel's new baby a kiss for me and Elsie a special hug from us both.

Love to all of you,
Ethel and Tom

Ethel looked forward to receiving letters from England. She savoured every word, reading them repeatedly. To each one she replied, telling her family about Canada, their flat, work and Tom's butcher store.

One morning during an early walk in the park, Tom turned to her with a proud look on his face, as if he had accomplished a great personal achievement. "I love Canada…especially the clean, fresh air. It makes breathing so much easier. I can even sigh deeply without coughing as much."

"And I'm so happy when you're happy," Ethel said. After they walked a ways in silence, she laughed out loud. "Maybe we can begin to think about another baby."

"I'd like that. It'd give our neighbours something different to talk about." He laughed and shifted his weight onto the other foot. "When there isn't any news of Elsie coming, their questions make me feel guilty." He laughed. "I always think they're waiting for me to tell them something that I don't even know myself."

"Unfair, isn't it?" Ethel said. "Surely they can figure out we'd bring her over if we could."

After such a conversation, Ethel always felt lonely for her family. As soon as they returned to the house, she sat down to write a letter.

They waited daily, but there was no word about Elsie being well enough to travel. Ethel worked at her jobs, made a few friends and thought a lot about her hometown of Enfield. Whenever she couldn't face another day without Elsie, she drew courage from writing to her.

Although their living quarters were modest, the small sheltered veranda offered a refreshing view of a park and proved to be a special place for Tom to sit. He got relief for his breathing, and Ethel often read to him from the newspaper.

"It's all coming together, luv. We have good people praying for us and helping things to happen," Tom said between coughs.

Ethel nodded. "But the most important part of our plan hasn't happened yet. Elsie hasn't joined us."

"I know, dear, but she's better off where she is…for the time being."

Tom's response surprised Ethel. The same conclusion said in different ways always ended their conversations. She hoped he wasn't giving up.

Through the fall and winter, Ethel monitored Tom's health, each day praying that his condition would lessen.

chapter nine

Bittersweet

Ethel grabbed the kitchen counter, afraid she would faint. This was the second time today that dizziness had caught her off guard.

"You're looking tired lately, luv." Tom put his arm around her as they sat on the couch.

"I've been feeling that way too," Ethel said, reaching for her knitting.

"Maybe you should go and see the doctor."

"I've never bothered to get one since I came to town. Just one of those details I haven't tended to." Ethel laughed.

"You can go and see my doctor. You like him, don't you?"

"Oh, I do." Ethel yawned. "I'll go by his office tomorrow on my way home from work."

Having made that decision, she picked up her knitting and continued to work on a sweater for a little girl who repeatedly came to the clinic without protection from the cold March winds.

The next night at suppertime, Ethel rushed in, laid a couple of parcels on the counter, sat down to face Tom and started to cry.

"What is it, Ethel?" he asked. "Did you go to the doctor's? Is that why you're upset? Did the doctor give you bad news?"

"I'm not upset." Ethel leaned over and hugged Tom. "We're going to have a baby."

"A baby? We are?" Tom's face lit up, his eyes bright with tears.

"Yes, in the fall…oh, Tom."

Tom stood and danced her around the room. "Perfect! Perfect timing!" He stopped and looked at her, "How far are you along?"

"More than two months, I figure. Oh, I should have been keeping track.

You know me and details lately. We must write to tell Elsie and Mum." She pushed the plates aside on the table. "Supper can wait. We just have to tell them, Tom."

> *March, 1912*
> *Dear Mum and Pa,*
> *Just a quick line. Thanks for reading my letters with Elsie, as well as all the care you give her. I'm so blessed to have you both. Please give our best to the family. We have such good news and want to share it. I just found out, I'm pregnant. My date is mid October or so. We are so happy.*
> *So a little more news while I have pencil in hand. Tom continues to do well in his meat store. He has many of the same customers returning two and three times a week for his special cuts. As I've probably mentioned, his store is close to our apartment, so he can come home to rest during the day if he needs to. And I meet the nicest people at the clinic. It's a fine job for me.*
> *You were right about this country being the wild and woolly west. You wouldn't have a hard time believing editorials in the newspapers about life out here, even though I wonder if they don't make some of it up just to create excitement. I cut some stories out to send to you.*
> *I read in the paper last week where they were asking British women not to come to Canada until this nation does more preparing for them. I believe most people think that being a man's wife and helper is the proper place for women. But there are some of us that think that women can do more things.*
> *I must go. Will write soon.*
> *I love you.*
> *Your daughter, Ethel*

It wasn't long before Ethel decided to help Tom in the butcher shop and gave in her notice. She liked the customers and enjoyed learning about their choices of meat. Some of the women lingered and talked about family issues or current wages, and some even asked for recipes. Ethel enjoyed their company.

Most of the time, she looked after keeping the shop tidy, shovelling the snow from the doorway and cleaning up Tom's back room. She cautioned herself against lifting anything heavy. "Taking care of us," she said and placed her hand across her waist.

The winter went quickly for Ethel, and she made many friends through the summer as she assisted Tom. Although she missed nursing at the clinic, she knew that she'd return later. Several times over the months, she'd had an opportunity to share her letters from home with other British people in her neighbourhood. The report was always heart-warming. She continually looked for Enfield news and familiar names from the newspapers sent over and shared them across the counter of Tom's butcher shop.

Looking at the calendar one fall morning, Ethel counted the days; the birth could happen anytime. Crossing her arms over her belly, she prayed, "Thank you, God, for remembering me." Ethel folded flannelette diapers onto a pile and placed them on the bed. The girls at work had given her blankets, a sweater set and a teddy bear. Part of her wanted this baby to be a little girl, but as she thought more about it, she knew Tom wanted a boy. William—Billie—would be good. Yes, after her father and brother. Surely Tom had a William in his family too. She'd ask him the next time they talked about names.

"Where do you want these potatoes?" Ethel heard her friendly neighbour's voice as Mrs. Farrow made her way into the kitchen.

"On the counter, please," Ethel called from the hall. "I'll be right there." Turning to Tom, who was busy hanging a picture, she said, "Tom, go and help Mrs. Farrow, would you please?"

Soon they were all sitting at the kitchen table, enjoying a festive goose dinner to which Mrs. Farrow had contributed several kinds of sweets. Over the last while, Ethel had been producing some tasty casseroles and main dishes with leftover cuts from the meat store. Several of the dishes had even caught the neighbour's eye, bringing many compliments for Ethel and her culinary talents.

"This goose from your shop, Tom?" Mrs. Farrow asked.

"It is—got a few fresh ones in yesterday. I saved the last one for our table; the rest went like hot cakes."

"I can see why." Looking over at Ethel, Mrs. Farrow asked, "And how are you feeling, Ethel?"

"Oh good, I guess, but I'll be glad when this baby's born."

"Ankles still swollen?"

"Not today."

Tom squirmed in his chair. "You didn't say anything about swollen ankles, luv."

"Every now and again they give me a bit of trouble. Nothing to worry about."

The meal continued with Ethel sharing Mum's news from Enfield. After dessert, Tom leaned back in his chair and said, "Between the two of you, this dinner would be the envy of half the people on the street."

They sat and talked until Mrs. Farrow began to pick up the dishes. "You don't have to cook and then clean up. Leave that for me," Tom said.

"That's very nice of you, Tom. In that case, I'll make my way home." She leaned over and hugged Ethel before walking towards the door. "You folks take care."

Tom cleared the table, and Ethel retired early to the bedroom. She hoped her time would come soon. She hadn't felt the same movement in the last few days, and it concerned her.

"How do you feel this morning, luv?" Tom asked, rousing her from her night's rest.

Ethel opened her eyes, stretched out her arms and sighed. "Too heavy…and full…too much of that tasty goose, I guess." Her feelings of anticipation for new life mixed with fear.

"You think it's getting your time?"

"I don't think it'll be long."

Ethel rested all day and the next one as well. That night, pains started in her lower back with steady contractions, and then toward morning, her water broke. Ethel started to time the pains.

"This is it, Tom. Go and fetch Mrs. Farrow and then bring the doctor."

Within a few minutes, Mrs. Farrow came in, excited and prepared to help.

Ethel's pains were now coming at two-minute intervals. "Six years since I've done this, Mrs. Farrow."

"No matter, the body don't forget."

"I'm starting to feel like I want to bear down," Ethel said, holding her breath, afraid that the baby was coming.

"You'd better wait until the doctor gets here."

"I can't. You'll have to deliver it. There's lots of hot water and towels in the kitchen. Ask Tom to show you. Go, bring them quick."

"If we're in this together, you better not do it on your own. I'll get things ready."

She came back, towels hanging over one arm and a pan of boiling water in her free hand, just as Ethel began to push.

"Hold on, Missus." The doctor rushed into the bedroom, threw his jacket on the chair and said, "Let me wash with some of that hot water before I catch this baby."

After drying his hands, he proceeded to examine Ethel. "It won't be long now, Mrs. Ayres. A few good pushes and you'll have yourself a baby."

Within moments, Ethel gave a long painful push, followed by an excruciating cry. She felt the baby slide from her body. Looking over the pillow she'd been clutching, she tried to see what was happening. Time seemed eternal. Quietness filled the room.

"Breathe, baby—cry!" Ethel agonized.

She looked at the doctor's face as he handed the baby to Mrs. Farrow, shaking his head. He came up to the bedside and reached for Ethel's hand. "I'm sorry, Mrs. Ayres. He...he was stillborn. There is nothing we can do."

"No! No! I don't believe you," Ethel wailed. "Oh, God, don't let this happen. It's too much for me. I can't lose this baby too."

"Bring Tom in," the doctor said to Mrs. Farrow. "I'll finish up here. She needs Tom to be with her now."

Within minutes, Tom came in and knelt at the side of the bed, resting his head on the pillow beside Ethel. "Oh luv, I'm so sorry. It's not fair."

"No, no, I won't believe it." Ethel tried to move away from Tom to see the baby.

"Here, Mrs. Ayres. Take this. It'll help you rest," the doctor said, handing her a glass of water and a pill.

"I don't want to rest. I want my Billie."

The doctor brought the baby to Ethel, wrapped in a blue blanket. "I'm sorry, Mrs. Ayres."

Ethel held the little bundle and then placed one hand on the baby's head as if to give a blessing. The doctor gently lifted the baby and walked away.

"We'll call the undertaker, and he'll look after everything," Tom said softly.

Ethel cried, covering her face with her hands and rocking her body back and forth.

The afternoon sun went down, and Tom continued to sit with Ethel, who refused tea and Mrs. Farrow's biscuits. The room grew dark, and Mrs. Farrow walked softly in and out of the bedroom, lighting the lamp, bringing Ethel a warm afghan and hot bricks for her feet. Ethel continued to sob deeply with throbbing shudders, refusing any comfort. The doctor came back, checked her and left. Tom and Mrs. Farrow watched her carefully, taking turns sitting with her.

The next morning, Tom sat down beside Ethel. "I went over to the undertaker's yesterday. I need to go back at one o'clock for the baby's burial. Is there anything you want me to do for you...for him?"

"No, Tom. I've been thinking, wondering. He wouldn't even know he was loved." She cried softly. "Children need to know they're wanted and loved. Billie died and never knew that."

"He knew, Ethel. You carried him with love, gave him your life, and shared your blood and your heartbeat. He knew." Tom paused. "Do you want me to take him the teddy bear?"

"No," Ethel spoke quickly. "I'd like to keep it." Reaching for Tom's hand, she continued, "Tom, do we have enough money? I mean for all the expenses." She closed her eyes and tried to speak between sobs. "This is something that you just don't save for."

Tom put his arm around her and held her close. "We'll get by, luv. Don't you worry."

Reaching for her Bible, she said, "Tom, would you take this and read Psalm 139 at the gravesite? Billie was 'fearfully and wonderfully made, knit together in his mother's womb,' and in God's eyes, he was perfect. He looked just like Elsie. I saw him, Tom. He was a big boy."

"I know, luv. I saw him too." They put their arms around each other.

Weeks passed before Ethel would even consider coming out of her bedroom except to use the washroom and take her bath. She took her meals beside her bed, and when Tom or Mrs. Farrow wanted to talk with her, they came into the bedroom.

"Don't you think you'd like to come out here and sit with me, luv?" Tom asked on a November morning. "There's some snow on the ground. It looks pretty. I thought that maybe I'd take you for a ride in that carriage that goes around the park. The sun's shining, and it's a beautiful day."

"I don't think so," Ethel said.

Tom sighed. "Well then, what would you like to do, because we're going to do something."

Ethel stared at Tom. "What did you say?"

"I said, 'We're going to do something.' I've tried, and you don't like any of my ideas. So you choose."

"I…I don't know what you mean," Ethel said.

"Ethel, you have to come out of this room. You will grieve Billy's death for a long time, but you don't have to do it in this room. I feel so alone. I lost a son too, you know."

Ethel looked at Tom, tears sliding down her face. "Oh, Tom, I'm so sorry. I didn't realize. I've been so selfish. Forgive me."

"I got pretty practiced at that over the last few weeks." He hugged her. "But enough is enough, and it's time you tried getting dressed and starting to do a bit."

"All right. I'll come out tomorrow, and maybe if the sun's shining, we'll go out on the veranda for a bit. Yes, I'd like that. Thanks for looking after me, Tom."

Ethel took the small teddy bear from her bed and placed it on the windowsill. "It's time we parted, Bear. Thanks for the company."

One of Ethel's first tasks now that she felt stronger was to write to Mum. She'd be wondering why there were no letters.

> November 1912
> Dear Mum,
> This is not going to be a long letter, but it's an important one for me to write. I'm sorry that I haven't written for a while, but Tom and I are grieving the death of a baby boy born on October 24th. We don't know why Billie died. The doctor said he was stillborn. Tom arranged for his burial. As you can imagine we are both heartbroken. But, gain some encouragement that by the time you receive this, we will be feeling somewhat better. Can you pass on this letter to Tom's father? And of course when the time is right, please tell Elsie. Our love to everyone.
> Ethel

Ethel felt badly that she hadn't had the fortitude to write this letter before now, but when completed, she felt an inner strength consume her.

Christmas came and went without much joy. The winter was fierce, and Ethel didn't venture far, except down the street to take over for Tom so he could rest. Several letters arrived from Elsie and Mum, as well as from the Ayres and other members of the Kemp family, offering words of sympathy.

Ethel regained her strength and began to think about applying for part-time work. There was no reason for her to stay at home, and it'd be good to get out among people again and to help financially.

When Tom came home one night after an exceptionally hard day, Ethel greeted him with her idea. "I'm thinking of applying for my old jobs, dear. Would that be all right with you?"

Tom smiled. "I think that's a very good idea."

"Good. I'll see about it in the morning."

They ate their supper, laughed and talked together as they used to, enjoying each other's company and teasing about Mrs. Farrow's upcoming pie contest.

It wasn't long before Ethel had both jobs secured, and she looked forward to renewing acquaintances. She purchased a new hat for Easter and suggested that she and Tom attend All Saints Anglican Church. "There's a speaker from England there who's going to remain following the service to talk to the congregation about women's votes. Can you imagine? I remember women back in London being thrown in jail for wanting the vote, and now the church is inviting someone from London to speak. Oh Tom, I wouldn't miss it for never."

One quiet Sunday morning late in May, Ethel woke up excited. "I'm feeling exceptionally good today. Something is going to happen for sure. Maybe it means Elsie's coming."

"Whatever are you talking about, luv?"

"I don't know, but I feel…well, we'll just wait and see," Ethel said.

Time passed, and Ethel kept teasing Tom that something was *in the air*, as she put it.

At suppertime, a couple of weeks later, she sat down very properly with hands in her lap and looked at Tom.

"What now, Ethel?" he said. "You look like the cat that just ran out the door with the canary."

"The cat ate the canary, Tom; he didn't run out the door. And besides, I don't want to talk about a cat or a canary; I want to talk about a baby."

"Aw, now, Ethel. You're not going to go back to that. You've been doing so good with your work and church and all."

"Tom." Ethel stood and looked down at him. "I'm going to have a baby I am. Oh Tom, I'm so happy. This time, well, this time it'll be different, I just know it."

"Do you mean it? Do you know for sure? When did you find out? When's he going to be born?"

"Yes, I mean it, and I know for sure. I found out today, and the doctor says February."

Ethel knew the good news of her pregnancy eased her grief somewhat for both the death of their son and their consistent disappointment about Elsie staying in England. Ethel immediately wrote to Elsie and her mother, telling them the wonderful news. Soon, she and Tom began to talk about being a family again.

The fall season gave way to an early snowfall in October. Another season of thanksgiving, and despite their memories of their loss last year, it was a joyful season. Snow fell across the yards like white sheets. Happy she'd taken a leave from her jobs again, she wouldn't have to walk on slippery streets.

Ethel felt the movement of her active baby and began to feel pressure in her lower back. Every day she thought about the delivery. Should she have a midwife and have her baby at home, or would she go to the hospital? She'd often wondered if it would have made a difference if she'd had Billie at the hospital. The doctor had said it wouldn't have mattered.

The excitement of their baby's arrival gave Christmas a new meaning. She remembered hearing conversations from different people on the immigration boat about wanting to be united with loved ones before Christmas. At that time, it had never occurred to Ethel that she might have several Christmas seasons before Elsie would join them. Worse still, she wondered how many more Christmas Days she'd have to endure missing her. With each one, Ethel had felt emptiness, a void, and this would be her fourth Christmas without her.

Tom was always attentive to the calendar and to the upcoming holiday. Early in the fall, he'd chosen a beautiful doll to send to Elsie with real looking hair and eyes that opened and closed. A yellow silk dress, accented with ribbon, gave the doll the appearance of an actual baby.

Ethel held the doll in her arms. "I remember when Elsie was this size. I can't imagine what it'd be like now to wrap my arms around her. I like to think of her playing with this doll, hugging it, being Mummy to it and telling it stories."

"I want Elsie to have her gift early, so she can look forward to opening it." Tom laid it in the box and closed the lid.

"You're so good to her, Tom," Ethel said. "She has come to know and love you through your letters and gifts. I can tell, the way she talks to you in her notes."

A perfect-sized tree in the corner of their living room stood boldly proclaiming the holy season. A few coloured candles clipped to the branch ends gave the tree a glow. Ethel had brought several family ornaments from home, and as she did every year when she put them on the tree, she told Tom their story. As usual, Ethel placed her father's hand-carved nativity scene in a visible place.

They decided to buy a few gifts with what little money they had left after paying their rent and getting groceries. "Life can't be all work," Ethel said. She liked a few surprises.

When Christmas morning arrived, Tom and Ethel went to their tree with a cup of tea and hot biscuits fresh from the oven. They were going to have a little time together, and then Mrs. Farrow would join them. Ethel gave Tom his present: two new cleavers.

"Beauties, they are, luv, thanks," Tom said. "Wherever did you get them? You couldn't have given me anything I needed more. And what's this?"

Ethel leaned across the arm of the chair and gave him a gift. "This one's from Elsie."

"Well, isn't she the clever one? She must have asked your mum to send our gifts separately, because I have one for you from her." Tom reached behind him and pulled out a gift wrapped with silver paper and handmade bows.

They both opened their gifts, wiping their eyes at the same time. Tom lifted his tie out first, and then Ethel unfolded a lovely silk scarf.

"We'll wear these all day. It'll be the next best thing to having Elsie with us," Ethel said.

They both donned their gifts, laughing together.

"Would you read me the card?" Ethel asked.

Tom opened the envelope that had arrived separate from the gifts, and a lock of hair fell out. They both reached for it at the same time.

"Oh, Tom," Ethel cried. "It's a curl. What a precious gift." Feeling its softness, she lifted it to her cheek. "I'll put it in a picture frame."

"Not for a while, I bet, you don't, luv."

"You're right. I just want to touch it and think of her." Ethel shifted toward Tom as he unfolded the card. "What did she say?"

November 1913
Enfield, England
Dear Mummy and Pa,
I hope you two like your gifts. I wanted to give you something for your neck so that when you put it on, you will think of me hugging you. I hope you're both well. I'm very excited about the baby. I hope it's a boy, and then you'll have one of each of us. Grandad is not always well. I read to him a lot now.
I love you both,
Elsie

"Elsie writes a good letter with your mother's help," Tom said and cleared his throat.

"She does indeed," Ethel said. "I must ask more about Pa the next time I write. It seems he's failing." Ethel gathered up some ribbon that had fallen from the table. "I wish we had a camera and could send some pictures to them."

Tom nodded. Christmas had always been special in their individual families in Enfield. She had memories of their folks visiting back and forth, sharing many homemade gifts of food and clothes. Tom's family was similar to hers in many ways, with neighbourhoods being close to each other, so they had combined the best from their individual traditions to create their own. She looked over at Elsie's picture, wondering if maybe next year they'd have a family Christmas with their new baby, and Elsie as well.

As Tom placed a long box on Ethel's knee, he said, "Here, luv, take a crack at this one."

"Thank you, Tom. Whatever could it be at this size?"

"Just open it up and you'll see. I know you won't get too much use out of it this time of year, but I remember seeing you soaking wet last summer."

She removed the paper. "I knew it'd be an umbrella. Oh, Tom, that's so thoughtful of you. And long winter gloves! They look so warm." Ethel pulled the gloves on and then reached over and hugged him. "I love them. Thank you so much. You are so dear to me. How can I begin to even the score?"

"You do every day, luv," he said. "Every day."

chapter ten

Time Moves On

Shifting her oversized body into a more comfortable position as she sat at the table with Tom on a Saturday morning, Ethel said, "Seems unlikely we'll get Elsie over for a while. I don't know how long this'll last." She handed the newspaper to Tom, pointing to the headlines:

"January 1914 opens a year of political and national unrest as the tension between countries grows and war becomes imminent."

"Not good news. It's hard enough for you being so far from Elsie and your family, isn't it? And with me being sick 'n all, and now this—"

"We're doing the best we can, Tom. I'm thankful for Mrs. Farrow; she's been a real treasure, keeping her eye on us both. Just like family." Ethel paused, reached down to rub her swollen ankle and continued, "Yes, it's been difficult at times, but we're managing."

After supper one stormy evening a month later, Ethel walked over to the end table and picked up Elsie's picture, obviously taken at a special occasion. A child's face with bright laughing eyes looked back at her. The dainty eyelet-trimmed collar on a white starched blouse encircled her neck and emphasized a tiny cross lying against the cotton. Elsie had one hand raised with a finger lifted, as if to get someone's attention.

"A beautiful smile, she has, that young one."

"She's got her mother's charm," Tom said.

"And her father's wit," Ethel added.

As Ethel stretched to place the picture back in its rightful position, a pain gripped her lower back, causing her to utter a sharp cry. "Oh Tom," she gasped for breath. "What an intense pain. Ah, another one; it's so deep in my back."

"Here, try to sit back; I'll go get Mrs. Farrow."

"No use doing that," Ethel said. "She's away. Went yesterday before the storm. Won't be back for two days. Her son came and got her."

"But she promised she'd be here when you needed her," Tom said, wringing his hands together. "You counted on her."

"She'd be here right now if she was next door waiting for this to happen. But I tell you, she's gone away with her son. I saw her go. And a good job she went when she did, because the snow hasn't let up all day."

"Well, maybe we should go to the hospital."

"Not tonight, we won't. Nothing was moving out there when I looked out the window a few hours ago. No, I'm going to have this baby right here. You and I can do it, if we have to."

"Now listen, there's nothing I wouldn't do for you," Tom said. "But deliver our baby? No! There's a limit."

"You don't have to deliver the baby. I'll just work along with my body. It knows what to do and when to do it and even how to do it." Ethel managed to smile.

"Now, Ethel," Tom said, "we could go to the hospital. Women do have babies there, you know, even in February snowstorms."

"Not this woman! We're not going out in this weather. No, Tom, and that's final."

"Ethel, I'm afraid," Tom said.

"I know, but we have to do what we can. I'll be fine. This time's different. I know it is."

"Maybe the pains will stop and we're worrying for nothing," Tom said. "We'll just wait."

"For what? Mrs. Farrow? Not a chance! I have a feeling this is the real thing. This baby's not going to wait for anybody."

Ethel and Tom spent the night preparing for the event that had already begun, while outside the snow swirled in circles. Towels filled the open surface of the side table, and water boiled on the stove. The sun rose on a new day after the storm, and Ethel waited.

A sharp knock at the door startled them both. Mrs. Farrow opened it and stuck her head into the room. "Thought I'd let you know I got back earlier than expected. My son brought me back as soon as the weather let up."

Tom jumped to his feet. "Are we glad to see you! Ethel went into labour last night about eleven o'clock. She figured by morning that we'd have us a baby. Come on in and take over. I might as well tell you, she doesn't want to go to the hospital."

Relieved and happy that her friend was back, Ethel continued to walk around their small rooms.

"I couldn't bear going to the hospital and labouring on my back," she said. "Why make him work uphill?"

"Don't worry," Mrs. Farrow soothed. "We'll talk to the doctor; maybe you'll be able to walk around while you wait. And you know Ma Nature well enough; she'll have her way. However, we *will* go to the hospital."

"I know the doctor is away, so we might have to take who we get." Ethel sensed the firmness in Mrs. Farrow's voice and conceded to her better judgment. "But all right, you win."

With some difficulty, Ethel delivered a baby boy an hour after they arrived. Mrs. Farrow stayed with her and listened to her grumble about the doctor. "He should have been working with me, asking me, coaching me, not ordering me around and telling me what to do and when to do it—as if my body didn't know the proper way."

Tom waited patiently in the hall, and when Ethel was prepared, Mrs. Farrow ushered him into the room.

"You've got a son," Ethel said proudly as Tom came up to the bed.

"And a good-sized one, they tell me," Tom answered. "How are you? Are you okay?"

"I'm fine. This new baby helps a lot." Ethel paused. "This is going to…"

"What, luv?" Tom asked, putting his hand on hers. "What are you trying to say?"

"It's just…my disappointment about…you know, Tom. It helps so much to hold a little one again." Remembering the birth of Elsie and Billie, she held this one close to her heart. "Raymond. Yes, we'll call him Raymond, just like you want. Oh, Tom, tell the neighbours so they won't worry."

Tom nodded his head. "I'll do that as soon as I go home." He kissed Ethel and said, "I know Raymond will bring us much happiness over the long winter months ahead. Somehow the talk of war in Europe seems far away when looking at the miracle of a newborn."

Summer brought a terrible fear of war. Ethel and Tom listened closely to as many radio broadcasts as they could.

"Turn it up, Tom. What'd he say?" asked Ethel as she listened to the announcer's voice over heavy static:

"On Tuesday, August 4, 1914, the world waits as England declares war on Germany. German troops have begun a long and arduous movement into Belgium, and Churchill has responded with a declaration: 'A state of war with Germany is at hand. The Germans approached the English Channel.'"

Ethel's original fears developed into trepidation. Tears ran down her cheeks. She looked away. *What about Elsie? Will I ever see her again? Will she and Mum and Pa be safe, and what about the young ones?*

The voice clattered on as Tom came and stood with Ethel:

"The opposing forces have broken through the Belgium resistance and continue to crush the front lines in Paris. They now look at England. Canada has joined hands with England, showing support, sending recruits, and organizing backup organizations to grow more wheat, roll more bandages, and work longer hours in factories."

Even though Ethel was far away from the home country, she felt a strong connection through obvious Canadian support. *But how does a woman give birth to a son and then find the courage to let him go off to war?* She couldn't bear to think of it.

Ethel's celebration of Raymond's birth transferred to concern for Tom as his coughing became more regular and his breathing problems worsened. His physical condition gradually deteriorated, and Ethel convinced him not to work any more. She secured her previous job at the clinic to help financially and shopped with great care, often making a soup bone and a few potatoes last a couple of meals. In addition, she always made sure Tom had his medicine.

In spite of his declining health, Ethel helped him to enjoy Raymond. He was a sociable child, capturing the attention of those close to him and holding it with his gestures. Tom enjoyed him and whenever possible entered into his playful activities. With some effort, he managed his letter-writing to Elsie. Ethel watched closely, comforting and encouraging him as she watched his fatigue grow through the year.

She was thankful that Mrs. Farrow kept near to them, often looking after both Tom and Raymond while Ethel worked. The doctor came to the flat regularly. His last test determined that Tom had heart trouble. Ethel was not surprised, since his condition had weakened over time.

With the additional stress of cardiac problems, Tom's breathing laboured. The doctor gave him a skin test and sent his sputum to the lab for diagnosis.

It seemed Elsie's letters were the best medicine for Tom. Ethel wiped away her tears as she read one to him.

October 1915
Dear Pa,

Thank you for all your letters. Even though you haven't written it, Gran thinks you're sick. I'm sorry about that. Mummy has helped me to know you, and I hope it's been the same for you. I've always enjoyed your letters. They mean so much to me. I think of you often and wish I could be with you, Mummy and Raymond. I was nine years old on my birthday, and school is going well. Gran reminded me this morning that miles do not change love. I like that. I was over to visit your family last week, and I passed on your letters.

I love you.
Elsie

In November, Tom began having severe coughing spells. He grew weaker over the next several weeks, and during one long night he slipped into a coma. Ethel held his hand until the end, wiping her tears, clearing her throat and speaking softly, assuring Tom of God's love. She talked quietly to him about how she'd care for Raymond and write to Elsie. Ethel was at his side in the flat he loved when he died as peacefully as he had lived.

Leaving the curtains drawn helped Ethel to shut out the morning sunshine. She couldn't bear the warm rays. Again she had a broken heart, but now Tom wasn't there to help her. She sat for a long while thinking of their life together. Grateful for their relationship, she knew he wouldn't have had as much time if they'd stayed in England. She looked at him and wiped her tears away. Then she crossed his hands over his waist and walked out of the room.

The doctor came and offered Ethel his condolences, did his paperwork and made the necessary arrangements. "I've put cardiac failure on his death registration because that was definitely the reason, but his lungs were tuberculoid as well. I think we should watch all of you over the next six months. Take the skin test; we don't want you sick," he said and then left the room.

When Raymond woke later that morning, Ethel cuddled him, knowing he was all she had. She told Mrs. Farrow later that day, "Tom looked at me for a long time and then said, 'Bye, Ethel. Keep lovin' us. I'm goin' on!' And then he took another shallow breath and smiled. Still with his eyes closed he said, 'Bye, Elsie, my little one. We *will* see each other.' He closed his eyes and within the hour had slipped into unconsciousness. Gentle, gracious, without fanfare. He just did it."

Several days later, Ethel sat down to pen a letter to Tom's family and then one to her mother. She wondered what words she could use to break the news and knew she couldn't say anything to make it easier, so she just began writing.

November 1915
Dear Mum and everybody,
This is one of the hardest letters I will ever write. As you know, Tom had become very sick over the last six months. He died this week. His last thoughts were of Elsie. I want her to know that he loved her very much and had hoped to be united with her. However, that will wait until eternity. Would you please tell her about Tom? I know you will be loving with her.

Doctor Austin told him that the fresh Canadian air would help. I'm sure it did, and it probably gave him more life than we are even aware. He enjoyed his butcher shop and the people who came to it—he at least realized his dream here in Canada.

So much has happened in these last five years: so much heartache and disappointment that it's hard to think. I'm very thankful for Raymond. I don't know what I'd do without him.

Mrs. Farrow continues to help me whenever I need her. She's God-sent. Please keep me in your prayers. I will write again soon. I love you and Pa, and I'm always thankful for you both being such loving grandparents to Elsie. I think of you often.
Ethel
P.S. I will write a letter to Elsie and mail it in a few days to follow yours.

Time Moves On

Ethel folded the letter and placed it in an envelope. She carefully counted enough pennies for a stamp and a loaf of bread and then bundled up Raymond and walked to the store.

Over the next while, Ethel watched Raymond and Mrs. Farrow for any symptoms of tuberculosis, but saw none. She arranged for all of them to have a skin test that proved they were free. What would she ever do if either one of them got sick?

"It's been three months now. You've got to get a hold of life again, Ethel." Mrs. Farrow's impatient voice rang through Ethel's head one day while they were having tea. "Your housework jobs aren't enough. You've got to learn to live again. You can't just sit here on poverty's doorstep and wait for the poorhouse to open its gates. It's time to move on."

"Move on to what?" Ethel asked. "My life, ever since I can remember, revolved around Tom." She started to shake with deep sobs. "I don't want to move on anywhere. I just want to miss him, think about him and cry for him. I've lost them both."

"What on earth do you mean, girl, you've lost them both?" Mrs. Farrow scolded.

"Both Elsie and Tom. She's going to be 10 years old. Her home is England. She'll not even want to come here. She's been with my parents longer than she was with me."

"Don't be silly. That kind of talk is just plain foolish. She hasn't forgotten who her mother is. I read that in her letters every time she writes."

"What's more," Ethel said, "how can I, a widow with a baby, ever hope to bring Elsie over here now? A world at war, her there and me here. And besides, I don't have any money. We were building up our savings, but with medical costs over the last few years, undertaker and cemetery expenses, well, we didn't even have enough as it was. My job barely keeps us out of the poorhouse—no more. It means starting all over again."

"All right then, when do you begin? You'll find a way. Now, don't be thinking on things that cause more trouble than you've already got."

With Mrs. Farrow's help, Ethel settled down and over the next year began to put life into perspective. Finding part-time work at the hospital and focusing on what needed to be done first, she prayed for the courage to step out and do it.

Continually thinking ahead for Raymond's sake, Ethel kept telling herself that he deserved everything that Tom would have provided for him. She continued to build on her plan, saving a little money every week, but she was easily discouraged. Seven years had now gone by since she'd come to Canada, and she admitted, there were days when she felt totally lost.

Weeks passed with no news from Elsie. Surely this had to mean good news, because for the most part, horrific news dominated. Then a short note came tucked in a hand-coloured card.

1917
Dear Mummy,
I hope you're getting along fine. Don't worry about us. We're doing okay. I hope you're not too lonely without Pa. I know it must be hard for you not knowing what's going on over here, but we feel safe in Enfield. I'm able to help Gran with the housework, especially since Grandad has started having dizzy spells. It takes both of them longer to do their chores. I say my prayers every night. Gran says the same moon smiles on you that looks over me.
Love Elsie

Ethel tucked the letter into an envelope. It sounded like both of her parents were slowing down. This had to be difficult for Elsie. What a gift she must be to them…strong, energetic and so caring.

Three days later German artillery bombarded the south of France. Attacks on London seemed relentless. The morning paper told the shocking news of bombings through the East End of London, hitting docks, train stations and schools—Enfield was north of London. Would it get worse?

Ethel heard nothing from Elsie over the next while. Then her letters began to flow in. She didn't often speak of her health. "We're still working at it, Mum, don't you worry none" was all she'd say. The letters spilled out experiences of danger and peril, stories of crowded bomb shelters and darkened windows. She wrote with an awareness of the evils of war, and her words expressed her fears.

A letter saying Elsie had been hit in the back with a piece of shrapnel while running to a shelter during an air raid caused Ethel additional concern. Elsie told her the pain of having it removed had been unbearable. But the surgery had been successful, and Elsie had recovered. "I think I'm going to be a nurse, Mum. They sure could have used some help when they were working on me."

Ethel always shared her news with Mrs. Farrow, but over time, she noticed inconsistencies in her neighbour's enthusiasm. Some days Elsie's letters would get her all fired up, as well as showing interest in Raymond's well-being; other times it took most of her energy just to get up in the morning. She'd been a good friend over the years and had helped Ethel through emotional turmoil while consistently introducing her to an independent Canadian lifestyle, for which she was thankful.

"Things are different here," Mrs. Farrow told Ethel one afternoon when she seemed to be feeling her old self. "Why, in Canada, you can make a difference. It's 1917, and that war isn't going to last forever. You can make a grand contribution to the Canadian life."

"But—a woman?"

"Nonsense! You know helping people is your first love," Mrs. Farrow said. "You've told me many times how you'd like to continue nursing—to be a midwife, open a clinic. And since you don't have your own little girl here in Canada, you'll bring them into the world for other women. You've worked when you needed to, ever since you came to Canada. I know you've little money, only enough to barely manage. Maybe I can help.

"You have to set your mind to do what you have to. Don't feel guilty about going out to work; you've got a family to raise. Why not go out into the country? People probably need you there even more. The flu's been raging, and it's leaving many folks on their backs."

"You're right," Ethel agreed as she set a teapot on the table. "I do love nursing. And I've always enjoyed helping women manage their pregnancies. Just to get them to work with their bodies to bring their little ones into the world is so rewarding. It's like experiencing birth again, isn't it? When I get excited about it, I can almost feel the labour pains." Ethel laughed.

"Yes, I have no doubt you've got what it takes to do what needs to be done. Can't beat that English blood. Good stock it is!" Mrs. Farrow teased. "Women are starting to be counted here in Canada. Go and add to the numbers."

"I admit I've noticed. And it appears to be happening in spite of resistance to women being out front and making decisions," Ethel added.

"But that's exactly what I mean. They're still doing it." Mrs. Farrow yawned, rubbed her eyes, and said, "Some people say it's only because the men are away to war and that somebody has to do it. But I think there's more to it than that. Women have come into their time."

"Nellie McClung among others have made a huge difference. She's concerned with important issues of women and children, temperance, even property issues regarding women's ownership."

"Come to think of it, I did read that women can own property. Perhaps that's stretching it a little far," Mrs. Farrow said thoughtfully.

"I don't know why owning property should become an issue," Ethel said. "Depending on the woman's circumstance, she should be able to make up her own mind. And women can vote now, at least here in Alberta." She poured hot tea into their cups. "I think Ontario women can vote in provincial elections as well this year, and that's a big change.

"Being able to own property would certainly make a difference in a lot of women's lives," Mrs. Farrow said, taking a sip of tea and placing the cup back in the saucer. "But voting—do you really think women across Canada will get the vote?"

"If McClung and her colleagues have their way, we'll all vote. And she also wants all the women who are raising children to have an allowance while their men are off to war."

"Sounds wonderful, but how far is she getting with it?" Mrs. Farrow asked. "We women have never had any power. That'd give us too much independence in some people's minds. There's a certain amount of responsibility that goes along with independence; I hope you young ones can handle it."

"We've had some pretty good models." Ethel laughed and moved closer to Mrs. Farrow. "Now enough of this serious talk. All of this must be tiring for you. Let's talk about the weather."

"Nonsense, I only get tired with work, not talk."

"I've made a nice casserole for supper tonight. Why don't you go and have a nap and then come back over and have a bite with us."

Mrs. Farrow left, and Ethel began to busy herself with the preparation of supper. When Raymond woke from his afternoon sleep, Ethel played with him on the floor. He was a delightful child, and he was learning to do many things. Ethel could see Tom's character already forming.

Picking up a newspaper from the table, Ethel glanced over the headlines. Stories of women and men dedicated to doing their part here and those committed to keeping Canada free on the front lines of the war zones filled the pages. Others, it seemed, stayed at home and learned needed skills in order to strengthen the Canada to which many would return.

A new urgency for peace seemed to invade people's hearts. The world had opened up through the lens of war, although it'd take generations to rebuild countries, as well as people's dreams. However, there were signs of leaders accepting responsibility to work with people in new ways. This was good news that Ethel followed with interest. She showed the paper to Mrs. Farrow later over dinner, and it created some good discussion.

Over the next few weeks, she talked to many people about the latest war news. Each day she read the daily newspaper and clipped out pictures and articles for future reference. She found it all interesting, although terribly stressful.

Ethel sat at the kitchen table, stunned beyond words. The coffee tasted bitter as she put the cup to her lips on that cloudy morning, and the heavy fragrance of the black syrup suited her mood. Word had just come to her that Mrs. Farrow was dead; a neighbour had found her lying on her kitchen floor. The doctor said a heart attack had taken her instantly. Ethel wished she hadn't died alone. Maybe if she'd been more attentive to Mrs. Farrow this wouldn't have happened. A woman who had given so much to others should have had someone with her in her final moments.

Again Ethel plunged into the grip of grief. Mrs. Farrow and Raymond had been the centre of her life since Tom's death, and now one of them was gone. Her death left Ethel lonely and sad. She felt cornered by circumstances beyond her control. Feeling homesick, she looked at her few pictures of British countryside and family members. Would she and Raymond stay in Canada with their remnant of life here? Did they have a choice?

As always, letters from home and daily newspapers provided an ongoing saga about the war. Ethel read that many people were talking about a ceasefire. Her hopes of travelling heightened. Rumours spread; sometimes she didn't know what to believe.

She sat down to consider her situation—could she afford tickets for her and Raymond to return to England? She went to her neighbours and asked to phone the train station for some information. The stationmaster bluntly said that she could travel to the east coast, but she should not plan passage to England at this time. It was unpredictable and very costly.

Overwhelming feelings of disappointment washed over her. She decided not to think about England until she could actually afford to make the arrangements.

Life in Canada had not turned out as she'd hoped. Ethel counted her bit of savings and wondered how long she could manage. She thought about moving; her apartment held too many sad memories. She struggled with loneliness, weighted down by her inability to make arrangements. She reasoned, planned and changed her mind, repeatedly. Each time she'd get her hopes up that she could go ahead, the common sense she prayed for would dash them.

Not often had she struggled with helplessness, but now it ruled her. She had no one with whom to discuss life. The few friends she'd made at the clinic and in her housework jobs were not close enough to know her personal struggle. She'd spent every free hour with Tom, and more lately with Raymond, and now her trusted friend, Mrs. Farrow, was gone.

She sat at her kitchen table and sobbed quietly while Raymond played on the floor at her feet. Then she took off her wedding band and put it on the ring finger of her right hand.

Oh God, what will I do? What a mess I'm in. How would Tom or I have any way of knowing our lives would end up like this? Is there any way for us to go forward?

Raising her head, she dried her tears and sat quietly for a long time. She thought about her parents in Enfield, Nurse Rankin, the hospital and, of course, Elsie. The telephone was becoming more popular, and Ethel had managed to talk to Elsie and to her mother. It would be encouraging to hear their voices, but she couldn't afford to pay for a call, so she picked up her trusted pen and paper. This had become her way of sharing her feelings of loss, as well as the good things that happened. She began a letter to Elsie, knowing Mum would read it.

Being careful not to say how hopeless she felt, she talked about her thoughts of returning to England and her growing belief that it was impossible. They'd understand, perhaps more than she did, how difficult transportation and money was to obtain during this war. They'd at least know that she was thinking of it.

"Come on, little man." Ethel picked up Raymond and cuddled him closely. "Writing that letter has given me new hope. You and your momma have some decisions to make. There are a few things we can't work out, but more that we can. So let's get at it. What do you think?"

He looked up at her with trusting eyes and stretched his arms around her neck. She stood and swung him around. Walking over to the window, she looked out for a long time, embracing him. "Nothing will ever separate me from you, son," she said.

What were her options? Everything that came to mind she immediately dismissed. Long quiet moments surrounded her and stilled her mind. Where was her courage? Over the years she'd lost some of the tenacity she had when she was younger. Perhaps it was fear of the unknown that kept her from stepping out in faith. But wasn't that what faith was, 'the substance of things hoped for, the evidence of things not seen'? That in itself was worth risking the safety of her four walls. She had to think beyond her immediate situation. She had to trust that God would continue to comfort her and give her assurance.

Ethel walked into her small kitchen and put on the kettle. Mum always said decisions were easier to make over a cup of tea. As she listened to the sizzle of the water heating, she began to think clearly. She poured the water into the teapot and sat down at the table with a cup and saucer. Looking into the empty cup, she knew that if she decided to fill it with the hot substance, it would be nurturing and tasty. If she made the decision to leave it in the teapot, she would remain thirsty. She filled the cup to the brim and then drank deeply.

Perhaps she'd take Mrs. Farrow's advice and accept some of those invitations she had received. Lillian, a distant relative who had settled in Edgerton, a rural area of Alberta, was anxious for Ethel to visit and, if possible, move there to begin a new life. It seemed so far away, but the more she considered the idea, the more possible it seemed. Surely she could do this. Yes, she'd take Raymond and move to the country.

After exchanging letters with Lillian, Ethel resigned from her job, put everything in order and prepared to travel out to the small town of Edgerton, approximately 150 miles southeast of Edmonton. She would raise her children there, Raymond now and Elsie when she came. They'd soon be a family again. There wouldn't be clinics or big hospitals in the country, so she might not be able to nurse. She'd start with housework and share her love for cooking.

After saying goodbye to her few friends in Edmonton, Ethel and Raymond travelled by train to Edgerton, a little town set in the sand hills. The rhythm of the wheels on the track brought back memories of travelling with Elsie, Mum, and Horace and then later from eastern Canada to Edmonton. Good memories, and she was going to make more.

PART III
1917-1920

chapter eleven

The People Find Ethel

Ethel decided on a house in Edgerton north of the bank, away from the centre of town and beside a row of willows. She was excited to have her own place. Grateful for Lillian's help when Ethel had moved from Edmonton, she was even more thankful for her financial assistance to rent this property. The house was large, comfortable and roomy. Windows on each side welcomed the sunshine, and a large veranda across the front of the house sheltered the front door from the winds.

One Saturday morning as she was putting her baking dishes away, a loud knock sounded on the side door.

"Good morning, Mrs. Ayres. Doc Smith's my name. Just wanted to come over and welcome you to our little town. Haven't been here long myself, and I hope you'll like it as much as I do."

The voice was exactly like the face: gentle and friendly, with a smile tucked under a broad moustache as he looked out from under a tweed peak cap. Holding a pipe in one hand, he leaned against the doorframe.

"Thank you, Doctor. I'm very glad to meet you. Would you come in?" Ethel asked.

"Don't mind if I do." He removed his hat. "Usually a little light on spare time, but I have a bit this morning."

Ethel had just made a pot of tea, so she poured the doctor a steaming cup and sat across the table from him.

"I was very happy to hear that you're a practical nurse." Doc Smith played with the stem of his pipe. "I hope you'll consider working with those of us on the front lines here in the district; there are some good nurses around."

"I've heard that, and I guess there's a great need."

"Yes, emotionally and physically. You'll soon learn that we're a community in grief, having said countless goodbyes. We have absent fathers and sons, empty chairs and broken hearts. The war's split families, spent lives, crushed dreams and left people reeling from its constant ravaging. And they said it would only last a few months." Clearing his throat, he continued, "Well, you know what grief is like. Lillian tells me you've had lots of it in your life."

"I have, Doctor, but I hope it's all behind me." Ethel changed the subject back. "The war cuts a wide swath, doesn't it? Men and women alike."

"Yes, I agree." He put his pipe in his pocket. "Families fear the worst as time goes on without word. Have you seen the Chauvin newspaper headlines this week? Men missing in action and killed in the line of duty—well, it mocks the sanctity of life."

"It does, and at the same time speaks of sacrifice and freedom." Ethel refilled his cup.

"We've had some husbands and sons return home without a limb, others with sickness needing family and community support to adjust and continue, while some have just left life behind and given up."

"They've gone through so much. It's hard to even imagine," Ethel said. "I guess those who couldn't go to war for one reason or another manage more than their share here on the home front."

"Absolutely! The war affects every generation; some wait, others move on, while a few give up and acknowledge the worst. There's closeness in this little town; we look after one another like family."

"It sounds as if I'll like it here."

"There's definitely a place for you. Many women have learned to work out of their home at jobs that men would ordinarily do, and some have trained for jobs both on the home front and beyond. Housewives are working in the fields, barns, factories, or wherever they're needed."

"I can see that people do what has to be done." Ethel took a drink of her tea. "Children grow up too fast in wartime, having to take responsibility before their time. Situations ordinarily managed by older family members get dumped in their lap."

"Yes, indeed," Doc Smith said. "And this flu. We can't seem to get ahead of it. It's a severe epidemic, attacking both the unhealthy and the strong, with a vengeance. Many people have died—young and old."

"So I've heard," Ethel said. "Let me know how I can help."

"I will, Mrs. Ayres. I hear you're a tremendous cook too, and there's always a need to make up meals for the families. Having a good cook and a good nurse in the community is a double benefit."

"And I enjoy being both." Ethel smoothed her apron with her hands.

"We go out when it's neither wheeling nor sleighing weather, but we make it through. In the winter we put our feet on hot bricks and wrap the big buffalo rug around us to keep warm."

"It sounds like quite an adventure," Ethel said.

"It is that, all right," the doctor said. "Butch Bonner usually drives, so we can concentrate on the patient we're going to see, rather than worrying about the driving. There've been many times in the winter when we couldn't see where the road was, but we kept going, just trusting God, our driver and the horse."

"Let's hope we don't have to worry about that weather for a while. I've had enough of winter for a few months," Ethel said.

"And it'll come soon enough," the doctor said. "Well, it's almost noon, and I've got three calls to make. I'd better go. And thanks for the tea."

The days cooled as the fall season settled. There'd even been a few snow flurries in the air. Ethel wondered how Elsie was. Maybe it was time for Ethel to pick up her pencil and write a letter.

> *October 1917*
> *Dear Elsie,*
>
> *How are you, dear? How's your school going? Thanks for sending me your recent story. It was very interesting. You're a good writer. Goodness, you're 11 years old now. Your grandmother says you are so pretty, and you are good company for her, Grandad and the young ones. Since she hasn't been feeling well, she appreciates your help so much. She tells me that you can bake wonderful biscuits. Good for you.*
>
> *Lillian Bonner has been very kind to me, opening up her home here in Edgerton, and then helping me move into my own place. It's nice and bright with lots of room.*
>
> *We're hearing in Canada that the war's almost over. You'll be glad when you don't have to run to shelters and cover your windows. Maybe there'll be an armistice soon. There've been so many lives lost on both sides. All of you have been so brave.*
>
> *I often think of your pa, Elsie. And when you come, I'll tell you about his life in Edmonton and the friends he made there. We'll go back and visit the people in our old building. They know you through your letters.*
>
> *Christmas is always a difficult season for me, but maybe being out here*

with some family will help. The sun is shining today, and I'm thankful for many things.

I'm sending your Christmas card and gift along with this letter so you'll get it in lots of time.

I love you.
Your mum

Time went by quickly, and Ethel immersed herself in the life of the small town. She made friends easily, and they helped her to fit into the community. Her first Christmas among the people turned into a blessing as neighbours invited her to their homes. She took advantage of the hymn-sing in front of the big Christmas tree and followed everybody inside for the hot chocolate and cookies the women had readied in the local church hall. The candles and excitement totally captured three-year-old Raymond. They went to all the Christmas events with Lillian, both in her home and around town. She introduced them to new people, giving them opportunity to respond to other invitations of hospitality.

Ethel met with St. Mary's Anglican congregation on Christmas Eve. The scent of candles and incense filled the space. It reminded her of St. Andrew's in Enfield and All Saints Church in Edmonton. As a widow with a small child, separated from her eldest child and extended family for seven long years and now struggling to find her place in a new community, she was very grateful that people had made room for her in their lives.

Yet, she seemed far removed from everybody tonight, even though people filled the seats around her. She looked at families sitting together. They'd go home to a Christmas tree and presents. They'd wake up tomorrow morning and begin their preparations for a family feast. And they'd gather around their big kitchen table and ask God's blessing together. She lowered her head and slowly turned the pages of the beloved prayer book. She knew the prayers by memory but still cherished the feel of the book in her hands. This particular one looked worn—a good sign of a faithful congregation.

Ethel had so many years of loss and grief. If only she could just leave all of it behind and start over. But could she do that? Did she want to do that? How would she fill the emptiness she felt?

The priest's soft voice brought her back to the moment as he led the people in the Christmas liturgy. She set aside her feelings of resentment and found his words comforting as she followed through the Scripture passages one by one as

The People Find Ethel

if she were the only one in the sanctuary. The candles burned brightly, reflecting a flickering image on the wall, and Ethel thought of how life could change just as quickly. The choir sang the carols with great fervour, and Ethel echoed every word in the quietness of her mind.

A young girl of about 12 years of age went to the lectern to read, and tears filled Ethel's eyes. Excitement carried the child's voice as she read the Christmas story—her face radiant, encircled by blonde hair caught up in ringlets. Ethel closed her eyes and thought about her younger sisters and Elsie. The old feelings of guilt and regret captured her when she thought how life might have been different if she'd remained in England. How often she'd fought those emotions; repeatedly they had rendered her helpless.

God, help me to remember everything good in the past, to count my blessings and look positively towards a new future in this town. Give me hope. Without that, I'm lost.

Ethel opened her eyes; the girl had finished her reading and was walking down the aisle towards her. She stopped at Ethel's pew and put out her hand. "Thank you for helping Mum, Mrs. Ayres. She's feeling much better now."

Just as quickly, the child moved to her own seat. After a few moments, Ethel turned her head to look back. Sitting beside her father and little brother, she lifted her hand, waving slightly. Obviously, her mother wasn't well enough to come to church, but perhaps she would be able to enjoy her family during Christmas.

After the service, some of the people decided to meet for breakfast in the morning before worship. "You come at eight o'clock, and there'll be a good old-fashioned western breakfast waiting for you," a man called out.

The next morning Ethel bundled up Raymond for the early walk to the church. After a hearty breakfast and lots of laughter, she carried the dishes back to the kitchen.

"We hope you're having a happy Christmas—maybe we can help to make it special for you," one of the women said.

"Thank you," Ethel replied. "It is a very good Christmas."

The long winter seemed to stretch out beyond the calendar months, bringing continued sickness with it such that Ethel had never seen in all her years of nursing. Besides the war devastating family life in so many ways, the dreaded influenza and gripe moved across the country, having no pity on size, age or gender, leaving those in its wake to bury the dead. Bad news caught Ethel off guard daily. People she'd come to know were among the deceased.

She started going out on some house calls with the doctor and was not surprised to discover a new excitement for nursing. Doctor Austin's words of encouragement about getting involved and finding her way echoed in her head.

"Oh, come on, Ethel," Lillian called to her one morning when she was shovelling the snow off the front steps. "You can't work all the time. Besides, I have someone I want you to meet. He's from England too, a veteran of the Boer War, in fact. You'll love his homeland stories. He's a gentle-natured man with the patience of Job and a good carpenter too—a handy man to have around. He fixed the cupboards down at the store in no time flat. Come on, he's over at the curling rink."

Wallace Bullymore leaned against the corner of a table and smiled as if he had a story to tell when Ethel walked into the room. He was tall and dark-haired with an appealing look as he bent over to pet his German shepherd. Ethel quickly appreciated his sense of humour and his careful speech.

She enjoyed his company, and within a month she invited him over to meet Raymond. She saw that he was a family man when he took to Raymond and asked her questions about Elsie and the family in England. There was a feeling of camaraderie between him and Raymond, which pleased Ethel. She needed to tell Elsie about this new relationship and hoped she'd approve.

April 1918
Dear Elsie,
We are hearing there will soon be a truce and the war will end. Thank God. It's been too long. I am very relieved that you have all been safe through this terrible time.

We're having a wonderful early spring—worth waiting for. I've never been so glad to see it as I was this year. The winter was long and cold on the prairies. I've surely not seen such storms. Having only known Canadian winters in Edmonton, I had no idea that weather could be as it is out here. I've learned many ways to get warm and stay that way.

We have much sickness both in town and in the rural areas. I go out to the homes sometimes with the local doctor if he needs some help. I like doing that and hope I can work more closely with him and the other nurses. There is so much need.

How are you getting along? Thanks for sending me your pictures and poems. I read one of your stories at the ladies meeting last night. They enjoyed it very much. Keep on writing. It tells me about you and your gentle ways.

Is your grandmother feeling any better? It sounds like her spells are getting closer together. Tell her I will get a letter off to her soon.

I've some wonderful news for you, Elsie. Lillian introduced me to a man who also came from England, so we have much in common. His name is Wallace Bullymore, and I think he will be a good friend. He and Raymond are already pals.

I will continue to plan for your trip to Canada. We must never give up, but you'll know when that time is right, dear. When you do come, it'll be out here to the country, but I'll be sure to take you to Edmonton to visit.

I love you,
Your mum

As spring continued to bring warm sunrays and fresh breezes, Ethel's relationship with Wallace grew. After spending considerable time with him, she decided to accept his invitation to share his life. As she reflected back over the worst winter weather she'd ever endured, she hoped the warm days would last forever, yet she knew that with winter would also come her December wedding. For this, she was thankful.

chapter twelve

Ethel: Prairie Nurse

One Monday morning, Ethel awakened early. The warm summer air gave way to a fresh new day. Her spirit echoed the familiar phrase "Behold, I make all things new" as she padded through the quiet house in her favourite slippers. Raymond was still sleeping, so she'd have an hour or so to herself.

The opportunity of beginning a new day—a new week—excited her. The hot morning tea satisfied her thirst and quieted her as she savoured each sip. Ethel liked Mondays; they motivated and challenged her and set her in motion. What would she do with this new day? She must choose carefully, for days without plans slip away.

A sudden knock broke into her thoughts. She opened the door, expecting to find a familiar face, but a rather timid, tired-looking woman stared up at her.

"Are you Mrs. Ayres? Ethel Ayres, the nurse? The midwife? I mean, do you deliver babies?" The woman's voice trembled. She wrung her hands nervously. Twice she looked over her shoulder to check the path behind her.

"I'm Mrs. Ayres. But, I don't deliver babies." Laughing a little, she continued, "The mother does that. I just catch them when nature does her work. Come in, won't you? How can I help you?" With a questioning glance, Ethel looked at the woman's midlife waist.

"No, ma'am, I won't bother you none. My name's Lottie. I live out in the South District. I just had to see for myself who was in town to look after me, if I got with child. Neighbours told me I might ask you."

"I think you should come on in, Lottie. We can't talk about this on the doorstep. Although the morning sun is lovely, it's not so nice standing here in the heat."

Ethel led Lottie into the kitchen and offered her a chair. "To answer your question, I'm a practical nurse, Lottie. I have my British certification of practical nursing. But I've some homework to do when the provincial accreditation is offered here in Alberta. Some of us are pretty excited about Alberta being among the five Canadian provinces to have registration legislated…so there'll be some new rules of admission and training, and of course, an examination for me."

"And in the meantime," Lottie said, "you can get lots of practice out here in the country."

"That's true. It seems to be working out that way, even though I thought I'd do housework and cooking when I came to town."

"But the rest of us can do that work. We can't do nursing. The word is out that people really like you. You care for them, and that shows when you nurse. I know some people who've changed their habits because of things they've learned from you."

"Thank you, Lottie. That's nice to hear."

"People gets used to living a certain way. They sometimes don't know what helps or hurts them. I heard you was talking to a farmer about eating all that fat on his meat. And he said it was his beast, he raised it and he was goin' to eat it." She lowered her voice. "I heard he told you that he was goin' to eat as much as he wanted; besides, the fat made it go down easy."

Ethel laughed. "I know who you're talking about. Did he tell you that I said that kind of eating would make *him* go down easy? If he's not careful, it'll be six feet down."

"Now we need to learn that kind of stuff. You make a lot of sense to me, Mrs. Ayres. I want you to be my nurse."

"There are a number of women in the area who already do this kind of nursing. One of them could be with you during your confinement and delivery," Ethel said. "I know that Nurse Sturgis is an excellent nurse. I'd recommend her to anyone. And you could always go to Mrs. Wolff's too. I'm sure there are others as well that I don't even know of."

"I know they're around, ma'am. And they're good. I know that for a fact."

"They have more recent experience in this kind of home-nursing than I do," Ethel added.

"Oh, I don't doubt that. I know they'd all be good or they wouldn't be doin' what they're doin'. But ma'am, if you pardon me for saying so, I'd like to make my plans with you. Everybody can have choice. And Ben and me, we talked and, well, will you be with me?"

"Lottie, you know something? Maybe you're the one to motivate me to write that examination. They sent me a letter a while back telling me it's coming. Years ago, I used to resent having to do it all over again, especially when I did so well on my exams in England. And then…so much happened in my life when I lived in Edmonton that I didn't get around to it, but now I feel privileged to be included in the registration."

"I'm happy to hear that. It'll take some pressure off some of the other women who help in the homes," Lottie said. "I know they're so busy."

Ethel paused for a moment. Looking closely at Lottie, Ethel asked, "Don't you think you're somewhat past that stage? Having a baby? I mean your age and all."

"I'm fifty years old, ma'am, or will be on my next birthday."

"Is this your first child?"

"No, Mrs. Ayres." Lottie paused, blinking her eyes until tears fell on her cheeks. "I gave birth to four healthy children many years ago." Her voice sunk into sobs. "Lost two more to a fire. I…I want a baby more than anything else in the world." Lottie wiped her tears away with her fingers. "And when I do get pregnant now, I just lose 'em. One right after another before their time."

Ethel moved toward her, placing her hand on the woman's shoulder. "Can you just love the ones you have and forget about having more?"

"No, ma'am. The living ones were taken away from me—not a nice story. We buried the other two on the hill. I don't expect you to understand. Ben don't understand either. Everybody tells me I need to go on in life. This is not about needin', it's about wantin'—wantin'!" Her voice grew louder, then broke off suddenly as she put her hands up on her face. "Why can't anybody see what I really want is to feel some peace? And I know best what I gotta do."

"I'm sorry, Lottie," Ethel said softly. "We need to talk some more."

"Mrs. Ayres, I just need to know one thing from you today, and then I'm goin'." Lottie looked down at her hands as she rubbed the arthritic knuckles. "If I get pregnant—will you look after me? I mean, come to the house and stay with me? Help me through the tough places. I heard you might do this."

Ethel thought ahead. She could do this. It was definitely something she wanted, and now this little woman was doing for her what she'd put off accepting for herself.

"Lottie, midwifery was my favourite part of nursing in England. I've worked with the best, and I'll be glad to get back to it," Ethel said. "Handing a mother her baby, well, that's got to be the most important gift of a lifetime. When you need me, I'll be here for you, I promise. But there are a lot of things you and I have to talk about before then."

"There's time for all that, but I got to go now, ma'am. I just had to hear you give your word. Real sorry to bother you. I'll be back." With that, Lottie got up, shook Ethel's hand and left. She walked down the path with a stride that looked like she had fire in the soles of her shoes.

Although the conversation only took 10 minutes, it kept Ethel thinking all day about this new beginning. She hadn't planned to go back to professional nursing so soon; frankly, she had wondered if it'd even be possible. Would this decision initiate more requests when the word got around the community? She hoped so!

Sitting at her kitchen table, Ethel thought about life. On this particular day, she looked through the window into a world where the sun constantly fought to warm the days after the summer's cool nights.

Raymond had just gone down for his nap, and Ethel decided to take the opportunity of a quiet hour to pen a letter to Elsie. She was painfully coming to the understanding that Elsie would come to Canada when she was able, and fretting would not make it happen sooner. She needed to find peace for herself in Elsie's decision. Maybe a letter would help.

> *July, 1918*
> *Dear Elsie: This is a quick note to say hello. I hope you and the family are doing well. Our spring was nice this year. But with very little rain so far, it's quite dry. I hope your grandparents are feeling better now that winter is over.*
>
> *Remember my friend Wallace? Well, some good news. We're making plans to be married later in December at Jim and Eunice Sawyer's house. They're good folks in the town who have become close friends to both of us. I'm starting to get excited about being a part of a new family circle, so I hope you are happy for me as I begin this new life. And, you'll like this, Wallace loves dogs. I've never had a dog, so that will be different for us.*
> *Write soon.*
> *Mum and Raymond*

When Raymond awoke, Ethel took him down to the post office to mail the letter, and then they went over to Bransgrove's Drugstore for ingredients to mix up some cough syrup. Isabelle, a friendly young girl with whom Ethel had spoken numerous times, came running up to them with pigtails bouncing on her back.

"Morning, Mrs. Ayres and Raymond." She knelt down and gave Raymond a hug.

"Good morning, Isabelle. Is your summer going well? I guess you'll be enjoying your holidays. It won't be long before you're back to school."

"I'm done." She twisted and turned with excitement.

"Oh? How old are you?" Ethel asked, admiring her auburn hair that framed her young face.

"Over 12, ma'am."

"All done school. Hmmm, are you sure?" Ethel knew this one was smart and wondered why she hadn't considered getting special training.

"Oh yes, ma'am. I'm going to get a job housekeeping."

"It sounds like you've made up your mind—for the present time anyway. I could use a little help with the house and with Raymond. Would you consider—"

"Thank you, ma'am. I'll go ask my mother and I'll run right over to tell you." She spun around and then ran down the path.

Isabelle was true to her word. In fact by the time Ethel returned home, Isabelle was already sitting on the front step, waiting for her. Yes, she could come. Later, Ethel sat down at the kitchen table to drink a mug of tea and eat her fresh cookies with Raymond. It would be nice to have Isabelle around the house.

The next day, Ethel picked up a letter from Elsie at the post office. The news about Ethel's mother was not good. She had begun to have numerous weak spells, and they were coming closer together. Elsie had a lot of support from friends and family, but Ethel could tell it was difficult for her. She was still attending school, but it sounded like she was very involved with her grandmother's ill health. This would naturally place a great burden on Elsie and Ethel's younger sisters who still lived at home.

After supper, Ethel brought it to Wallace's attention. They read the letter again. Wallace commented on Elsie's strength of character. Ethel's deep sorrow about her mother's sickness, mixed with an overwhelming sense of gratitude that she had given Elsie such a good home, brought her to tears.

chapter thirteen

Awakened to Need

Bang! Bang! Rain lashed against the windowpanes, hammering out a constant rhythm. Under the fall storm's wrath, wind pushed branches against the window while, against the backdrop of the velvet night sky, silver streaks of lightning stabbed the darkness.

Again Ethel heard a bang. Was that back door loose? She knew she had locked it with her own hands. She settled again into her soft lilac-scented pillow and wondered about the women who were due to deliver. Some lived in town, and others were miles out in the country. She couldn't bring herself to think about the condition of the roads in this rain, let alone the task of driving on them. She hoped this was not the reason for disrupting her sleep. It wouldn't be the doctor, or she'd hear him hollering and pounding loud enough to wake her and the neighbours.

Wait. What was that? She listened again. A voice? No, she must be dreaming. Ethel opened her eyes and glanced around the room. She grew uneasy. The storm had darkened the sky so much that it was difficult to know how close it actually was to dawn.

She edged out of bed, reached for her housecoat and moved her feet over the wooden floor, feeling for her slippers. She groped for the oil lamp, found it on the bureau and lit it. The light cast a soft glow on the shiny pine floor as she made her way down the hall past several closed doors, including Isabelle's, who had stayed over to help with extra cleaning.

Ethel carried the lamp through her parlour, feeling the softness of hand-sewn rugs underfoot. She walked over to the kitchen wood-box, picked up a short log and stuck it into the dying flames. Cold winds last night had caused her to put a fire in the wood stove, for which she was grateful.

A bang on the door made her turn. Crossing the room quickly, she flung open the door and saw a young girl's face.

"Tina, Tina! Oh my, child! What are you doing here? Come on, we'll get you into the house." Ethel gathered Tina in her arms and moved back into the room. She saw fear. Her eyes, red from crying, focused directly on Ethel.

"Oh, Mrs. Ayres, please come to my momma," she cried. "When I left the house, she was real bad."

"What's the matter with her, luv?"

"I don't know, ma'am. She was throwing up and then she started gagging. Then she got so weak she couldn't even do that anymore."

"Goodness, child, warm yourself up while I get ready," she said.

Ethel remembered seeing the Pattersons when they'd come into town for supplies, but Molly Patterson's sickness was news to her. It hadn't been too long ago that Mr. Patterson had died from a bush accident, so there would be just Tina and her mother on the farm.

Ethel thought about the slough and remembered how the water easily flooded over the road. It was a narrow trek, low land, mucky and wet at the driest of times. It could be impassable during rainstorms.

Promising they'd soon be on their way, Ethel checked her supplies. The remedy cupboard opened easily, and she surveyed a colourful collection of bottles and tins. A weakened area at the top of the hot water bottle reminded her to go to Charlie Bransgrove's drugstore and buy a new one when she came back from the country. After making her selections, she went into the bedroom to wake Isabelle and tell her she'd be away most of the day. If she needed help with Raymond, Lillian would be handy.

Ethel returned to the kitchen carrying a jacket and overalls. "We'll go and ask Butch to take us out with Ol' Dick. Butch rather likes the challenge of driving in the country, and he won't mind this weather. Come on, put on these dry clothes and then we'll go. Thank goodness, it's stopped raining."

Ethel and Tina went over to the Bonners. The kitchen light burned brightly. Opening the door a bit, Ethel called, "Butch, are you up?"

"Yeah, I'm up. Quite a morning for you to come visiting," he teased.

"I've got to go out the south road. Molly Patterson's sick. Want to drive Ol' Dick out for us?"

Butch pushed the door open with his boot, laces dragging on the floor. "That should be quite a ride after a night like this one. Just give me a minute and I'll be with you."

Ten minutes later, they began the trek leading away from town. Splashing the water as he put one hoof in front of the other, the horse lunged forward, trying to keep his footing. Suddenly, with a jarring lurch, the buggy stopped.

"No, Ol' Dick! Keep us moving, boy." Butch lifted the reins high and slapped the horse's back. "Giddy-up. Go on, Ol' Dick. Come on, boy, take us through here. Go!"

The horse strained and pulled, trying to obey the command, but the sand was too deep, sloppy and heavy. Slowly, it reached the wheel hubs and piled up around the axle.

"Come on, Tina 'n Ethel, we gotta get out. I'll lead Ol' Dick through," Butch said. Tina began to cry softly.

"We'll be all right." Ethel put her arm around Tina. "The water's not deep. It'll only take a little longer." Ethel's voice was soft and gentle, without fear. "When we get through the worst of it, we can climb back into the buggy."

All at once, Ethel's feet went out from underneath her, and down she went—face first. What a soupy mess. The gritty sand seeped between her lips. Her arms flailing, she managed to stand up and grasp the side of the buggy again. Wet and mucky, she lifted one heavy boot after the other to gain her balance. She wiped her mouth and rubbed her hands against her chest.

When Ol' Dick finally managed to get the buggy up on dry ground, Ethel helped Tina climb back inside, and Butch led the horse. The little homestead lovingly built by Mr. Patterson came into view straight ahead of them.

Ethel and Tina struggled out of their muddy boots and overalls and left them on the porch. They entered the cabin and walked across the room. Through the shadows, Ethel noticed two beds standing in the corner of the room.

"Come over to the basin and we'll wash up," Ethel said.

When they had dried their hands and tidied themselves, Tina quickly climbed up on one of the beds. "Momma! I'm here, Momma! Mrs. Ayres is here too. Oh Momma, please answer me."

Ethel folded the covers back. "Mrs. Patterson, can you hear me? Can you open your eyes?"

Molly Patterson lay as still as death itself. Her hair spread over the cream-coloured pillow; her pale cheeks and dry lips appeared void of life. Ethel looked at her face—long eyelashes prevented anyone from looking into her world.

Ethel took one of her hands and lifted the back of it to her own face. Molly's dry skin was hot, and her chest moved in shallow breaths. The ripe sweet odour of her breath permeated the stagnant air between her and Ethel.

"Is she dead, Mrs. Ayres? Is she dead?" Tina sobbed, reaching for her mother's hand.

For a moment, Ethel didn't answer. Then she put one arm around Tina and kissed her forehead. "No, dear, but you're right. Your momma's very sick."

Ethel turned back to Molly and wiped her brow. The extreme heat of her body and dryness of her lips and mouth indicated that Molly had a very high fever. Lots of liquids and wet cloths might break it. A little safflower, ginger or rosehip brewed into tea and sweetened with honey might be the answer—anything to make her perspire.

"Better go out and tell Butch to let Isabelle know I'll be a while. Tell him to come back tomorrow evening after supper," Ethel instructed Tina.

Ethel pulled her pocket watch from its pouch to take Molly's pulse. Startled, she realized the watch had stopped. "I'm sure I wound it. I'm always so careful." As her eyes focused on its face, she saw hairline sketches across the glass and realized, with a stab of grief, it must have gotten wet when she fell. Through the years, the watch had been a constant reminder of her father's confidence.

The hands on the big clock on the hearth moved slowly—two hours, then three. Ethel noticed Tina watching with a worried look.

Ethel bathed Molly again, hoping the water would be comforting. Tina continued to bring tea. She whispered gently, "Open your mouth, Momma. Take a few sips. Please, Momma."

Slowly over time, Molly's lips parted and she sipped the herbal liquid. Through the night, she began to drink more liquids and move around in the bed. Ethel changed her nightdress and washed her hands and face while talking softly to her.

The following morning, the sun streamed through the window, spilling warmth into the room. Ethel put another pillow behind Molly's head to lift her up a little and could see she was awake and aware of what was going on.

"I'm glad you're feeling better. You had us worried yesterday," Ethel said.

"When did you come out?" Molly asked weakly.

"Tina was at my place before the sun was up yesterday morning."

"How'd you ever do it?" she asked Tina in a faint voice.

"I got wet and muddy, but I asked Mrs. Ayres to come."

During the day, weariness gripped Ethel, as she'd only had short rest times, but she persevered to work alongside Tina to prepare food to store in the cold room. They baked bread and made potato scones. Ethel could see that Tina, with her fast and efficient manner, could look after Molly. She reminded Ethel of the precious relationship between a 12-year-old girl and her mother.

"You're an angel of mercy, Mrs. Ayres," Molly said as Ethel prepared to leave later in the day.

"Tut, tut, I didn't do anything for you that you wouldn't do for me," Ethel replied. "People need people, that's all. Often, someone comes looking for a word of advice or a remedy of some sort, maybe a poultice or liniment and cough syrup. And when I need something, they're always there for me."

Ethel gave Tina final instructions just as Butch arrived to pick her up. She stepped into the buggy and waved goodbye. Butch turned Ol' Dick north toward town. As she settled, Ethel thought about Isabelle and Raymond and hoped they'd gotten along all right.

Angel of mercy! A smile crossed Ethel's face. A comfortable feeling filled her. She didn't look for compliments, but it felt good to hear one. As she jiggled along in the buggy, she looked over the fields and trees, which had already changed to their autumn colours.

"I know you've been out and about a lot this fall," Butch said as he glanced at Ethel. "Are you going to cook your beau a harvest dinner?"

Ethel chuckled at Butch's description of Wallace's relationship with her. "Can't promise," Ethel replied. "But, I'll be sure to make him a goose sandwich if we can't get together for a meal." Hearing of three more bouts of flu, Ethel knew she shouldn't even promise that.

Butch drove the horse up to the front of her house, and Ethel thanked him for coming out to get her. She picked up her bag and stepped down. "I really appreciate you, Butch; you know that, don't you? Whatever would I do without you? Thanks again. Just put it on my tab. And by the way, it's going to get pretty big if you never collect."

"Nah, I'm not going to collect. You know me—I'm always glad to help, Ethel. Come and get me anytime. I'll go put Ol' Dick away now." With that, he drove toward his barn.

chapter fourteen

Bad News—Good News

Early in the day, Ethel began to prepare food for company. Pots and pans were piled together, spoons and knives laid across the sideboard as if resting from a big job.

"What a mess! This reminds me of our kitchen at home in Enfield, Isabelle." Ethel grinned at her young partner. "When our big family gathered for a special dinner, there'd be such disorder and laughter." She paused and then said, "And it was always such a happy time."

"I like to hear your stories of England, Mrs. Ayres," Isabelle said.

"It's a grand place." Ethel gathered a few crumbs from the kitchen table, where they'd been preparing the food. "My family's pretty small over here in comparison to Mum's family, but I still manage to create as much chaos as she did."

Later in the day, Ethel welcomed Wallace along with the Bonners. Ethel settled them with tea, scones and fresh jam in her living room. "Come on, Isabelle," Ethel said. "We'll set everything out. I missed having a harvest dinner this year. Since the first snow fell today, maybe we can celebrate that."

They both laughed at the thought of celebrating a snowfall and commented that by the middle of winter they'd be complaining about it.

After a delicious meal, the women washed the dishes and put them away. Ethel brought out the dominoes as well as the cribbage board and placed them on the table.

"Come on, let's test your skill," she invited her guests. Laughter and jokes accompanied the games, and they soon spent the evening.

Lillian and her family said their goodbyes, leaving Ethel and Wallace to tidy up. Isabelle had planned to spend the night, so she went upstairs with Raymond, promising to read him his favourite story before he went to sleep.

"That was a wonderful meal, Ethel," Wallace said as he sat down beside her. He reached for her hand and said, "I've been holding something back all night, I'm afraid."

"Oh? What's that? You had that extra piece of pie when my back was turned?" Ethel teased.

"That too," Wallace said. "Ethel, I have some very bad news. I didn't want to tell you until after your party tonight. But…your sister Florence wrote me a note and asked me to tell you that—"

"My sister wrote to you? Whatever would she write you a letter for? She doesn't even know you. My goodness, what did she say?"

"That's what I'm getting to," Wallace said. "Florence said she didn't want you to read this when you were alone, so she addressed it to me to give to you." Wallace searched in his sweater pocket and pulled out a piece of paper, carefully unfolded it and handed it to Ethel.

Reaching out for it, she stared at Wallace. "Is it Elsie, luv?"

"No, it's not Elsie. It's your mum. I'm so sorry, Ethel."

Quickly Ethel looked down at the letter and scanned for the dreaded words:

Mum passed today—October 25th. I was at her bedside. I'm sorry to tell you this news. We were all thinking Pa would be the first to go and that Mum was stronger. But her lungs weakened and pneumonia set in. She was just fifty-six years old. Thank you for leaving Elsie with her and Pa. She was such a good little trooper through it all and has been a great friend to the young ones. We will have a nice service for Mum at the church, and I'm so thankful that Pa will be able to attend. Those two had a special love for each other. I hope he can rally now—without Mum, that is. I will write again after things settle down.

Love always,
Florence

"Mum's gone? It's so hard to believe." Ethel sobbed and leaned over the table. "And now I suppose Elsie and the girls will care for Pa. My, what a responsibility for them."

"It sounds like Elsie's been a big help to the family," Wallace said.

"And now Mum won't be there to help her think things through," Ethel said.

"No luv," Wallace said quietly. "Your mum's not there any more."

"Thank you for staying, Wallace, while I read this. It helps," Ethel said softly. "I'm afraid I have to ask you to let yourself out now. It seems I can't think anymore. I'm rather spent. I just want to go to my bed."

They sat together in silence for a few moments, and then Wallace reached over and hugged her.

"I understand. Let Isabelle get up with Raymond in the morning and you rest. I'll drop in later in the day and see how you are. And, Ethel, if you need anything, don't hesitate to ask."

"Thank you, I won't."

She continued to sit at the table and turn the letter over in her fingers. Finally turning the wick down in the lamp, she extinguished the light and invited darkness to invade the kitchen. The peace for which she yearned was not within reach.

The ceasefire happened, and finally the word that everyone was waiting for came. The war was over! November 11th marked the date. Ethel and Wallace sat listening to the broadcast through a static-filled station. They welcomed the news with great fervour.

Wallace had served in the Boer War, and although he didn't talk much about it, Ethel knew he'd remember the feeling of coming home. Joy filled Ethel as she thought of the men and women returning. The town mourned its losses—now they were dancing in the streets for the living. The condolences people had offered to her about her mother's death had helped Ethel enormously, but the news about the war helped even more.

Ethel sat in her church pew on Sunday morning, going early to pray. She felt the excitement in people's chatter and laughter as they gathered. The priest spoke during his sermon of rebuilding the country as well as strengthening people's lives with God's help. Ethel left the service feeling that new life would begin with this armistice. Politicians had already announced great plans for building the country's economy. Men and women would be returning home from war looking for work, renewing relationships and arranging family reunions. Hopefully, they would pack church pews to overflowing again and sing songs of thanksgiving. Oh, it would be such a celebration of new life!

Ethel stood in front of the post office after retrieving a letter from England and several Christmas cards. Her sister Mabel's name and address clearly printed in the upper left-hand corner and her usual scroll to Mrs. E. Ayres across the middle of the envelope made Ethel cautious. Slowly she peeled back the lip and slid out the letter.

Dear Sis:
It is with much sadness that I tell you that Pa died early last week with his kidney trouble—November 17th. I was with him to say goodbye.

Ethel closed the letter and blinked away the tears. She thought for a minute she'd have to sit down. Taking a deep breath, she opened the sheet of paper again and continued slowly.

Elsie and the girls were so good to both Mum and Pa in those last days, you'd be proud of them. They made a regular little team. We had a nice service for Pa at the church. May he rest in peace. Many of his fellow labourers came to pay their respects. We were greatly encouraged. I will write soon.
Love, Mabel

She had expected the news of one death because of past letters, but not both—and not so close together. It was sad they'd died within weeks of one another. Yet, they'd lived that way. Pa couldn't go on in life without his Beth. She thought about his gentle-nature—always with a word of encouragement and a little story to go with it. Wallace reminded her in some ways of Pa.

Wallace! Wedding! What would she do? Just days before her wedding date! With her heavy heart, Ethel couldn't imagine feeling the joy of the occasion.

After considerable thought and in spite of her grief, Ethel continued as planned with her marriage to Wallace. Mum and Pa had been so pleased that she had found happiness again; she needed to proceed with her plans.

Excitement built in the community as Ethel and Wallace's wedding date drew closer. People gave gifts and cards, and the announcement in the paper told bits of their individual histories before coming to Edgerton.

"Your plans are coming together nicely, Mrs. Ayres. I'm happy for you," the priest said to Ethel when she shook hands with him on the morning he'd read the bans in church.

"Yes, despite all my bad news lately, something very good is about to happen."

Wallace caught up to Ethel as she walked down the steps. "Let's go over to the Cozy Café for lunch. Maybe there'll be some of that homemade soup left over for us."

Ethel looked down at her hand, thought of hearing their names read in church, and rubbed her empty ring finger with her thumb. How nice it would be to see a ring on it again. "Yes, let's go. We have something to celebrate today."

chapter fifteen

Picking Up the Pace

Red ribbons and cedar boughs decorated the living room at the Sawyers' house in preparation for the wedding. Ethel and Wallace said their vows one month and one day after the armistice and in the midst of the tremendous grief over the death of both of Ethel's parents. Ethel liked to think of her courage to go ahead with her wedding as symbolic, in some way, of her parents' strong love for each other.

Pictures of Elsie and other members of both families sat on the Sawyers' sideboard as if to encourage Ethel on this special day. She knew that this was the best decision she'd made in a long time; she cherished Wallace and the promise of their life together.

People brought in baked goods and placed them on the sideboard alongside the photographs. A neighbour served a wonderful meal of roast beef with browned potatoes and carrots, with side dishes of coleslaw and pickles. Apple pie and cheese slices sat on the counter along with cookies, squares and tarts. It was truly a feast.

"We'll do this every year to celebrate this occasion if we get fed like this," Jim Sawyer said.

"I don't think we'd get away with it," Wallace said.

"I meant the meal, not the wedding," Jim said. And everybody laughed.

Later that night, Ethel hugged Wallace and said, "This feels so right. Not just because of the wedding, but because we both need something good in our lives."

"I'm glad you feel that way, Mrs. Bullymore, because it's for a lifetime." He returned her hug.

They both tucked Raymond into bed later that night, and Ethel marvelled at how well he had adjusted to having Wallace in and out of the house over the last while. He showed love for Wallace already, and now that they were a family, they'd have lots of time to develop a deep relationship with each other.

"Goodnight, dear," Ethel said to Raymond.

"Have a good sleep, son," Wallace said softly. "It's been a big day. We're going to turn this lamp down and leave the door open for you."

How Ethel loved that little boy. He was four years old and had a big adjustment to make in his life, again. But he could do it…children could. Elsie had proven that. She had lost her mother to Canada at that age, and Raymond had gained a father.

Ethel walked over to the sideboard and picked up a letter from Elsie that Wallace had just brought in. She read quickly until she got to the part about Mum.

> *I know you will mourn Gran and Grandad and especially miss writing to Gran. She didn't want me to tell you that she was getting weak. Aunt Mabel called it "failing." I noticed it more every day. She'd never been right since that bad spell a while back. I don't want you to be too sad, because she often talked about going home to be with Jesus. She wanted me to go to Canada if anything happened to her. She even put money away for me and has been very generous to me over time, teasing me to put it to a good use. I cared for her the best I could and believe I was a comfort. Now I'll continue with my schooling until the time seems right for me to come and join you. My "little aunts" as I tease Evelyn and Eleanor are my very best friends. I will miss them terribly when I come to Canada.*

"When I come to Canada." Ethel's heart warmed as she read her letter, even with the sad news of Mum's poor health before she died. She had planted the idea in Elsie's mind about coming to Canada. Ethel tried to picture Mum in her mind, but it was difficult; it had been so long. She wept at the words of her mother's ill health and prayed she hadn't suffered.

"News from England?" Wallace asked, hanging his coat on the rack. He sat down, acknowledging his dog with a pat.

"Some good and some not so good," Ethel answered. "Elsie mentioned coming to Canada. This is good news. And she talked about Mum's health toward the end—how she didn't want anybody to tell me she was failing."

"I can understand that," Wallace said. "It didn't surprise me that Elsie would see her grandparents through to their death."

Picking Up the Pace

"I agree. Mum mothered and grandmothered her," Ethel said thoughtfully as she folded the letter and put it at the back of the pile of wedding congratulations. "And for that I'm thankful. Elsie sounds so mature for her age; it shows in her letters. I wonder if she'll really come over."

"We'll wait and see," Wallace said, "But I'd be willing to bet you a supper at the Cozy that she comes when she finishes school. She's only 12 and has some growing up to do. It's probably better for her to bring certain things to an end."

Ethel knew Wallace was right. She was well practiced at waiting.

It seemed like the wedding celebration and the Christmas season melted into one, and soon Ethel hung the mistletoe for New Year's Eve.

The Brown house, as the Edgerton folks affectionately called it, was spacious, and Ethel and Wallace hadn't lived there long before they decided to make better use of the rooms. Wallace worked as custodian in the bank and often said that employees and other people needed room and board. So they opened the house for boarders, and Ethel used her homemaking and cooking skills. She continued her nursing whenever an opportunity opened to her.

Now that the war over, Ethel began to think of ways to encourage people. She made some New Year's resolutions and set several goals. To write her nursing registration examinations and do some long overdue redecorating were foremost on her list. And wouldn't another baby be nice!

Her constant yearning to bring Elsie to Canada eased. She had some peace in knowing Elsie would come when she was ready. She had a good life established in Enfield with school, friends and family. It wasn't fair to disrupt what Mum had helped her create. Elsie would be 13 this year, and Ethel thought that the timing of any future reunion should be left in her hands. Now that both Mum and Pa were gone, Elsie would have to decide what she wanted to do.

In those difficult early days, the thought of Elsie coming had given Ethel hope. But now she needed to honour Elsie's wishes and focus on her own life. As well, Ethel knew returning to England was not an option now. Ethel walked into the kitchen as Wallace stuffed wood into the stove. "I'm going to apply for my Canadian nursing license this year, Wallace."

"You're going to do what?" he asked as he put the lid back on the stove to settle the licking flames.

"Apply for my nursing registration. Write the examination set by the University of Alberta; I really need to do it. It gives my nursing more credibility, and I'll get a Canadian certificate."

"Well, it's about time, I might say. There's been some talk about it in the papers, and I've been wondering when you'd do it."

"I have some catching up to do, but I'm sure I won't have any problem. I'll have to go into Edmonton to write it."

"We'll manage. The folks just love to have an opportunity to pay us back for all the good work you've done among them."

"They're more than generous, both with their pocketbooks and their love." Ethel dumped a half pail of wrinkled carrots into a wooden bowl and poured on some water to prepare them. The large cooking onions that had brought tears to her eyes earlier as she'd peeled them lay on the cutting board, and the cubed potatoes simmered in a rich beef broth saved from last night's dinner. She wondered about dumplings and knew they'd look nice puffed up on top of the stew but decided against them because of the time.

Doc Smith had arranged for Butch Bonner to pick up some food and deliver it to families who suffered with influenza. Ethel knew that children in both those kitchens would be waiting to pull a chair up to the table, and her stew would make a good meal for any who still had an appetite. She dumped the ingredients together in her big pot, stirred them with a wooden spoon and set the pot on the front of the stove. Then she hurried into the back room to finish her washing.

After a pleasant morning's work, Ethel and Wallace sat down to dinner. She served up two bowls of stew before putting on the lid and setting two pots outside on the back step ready for Butch.

Looking out the kitchen window, Ethel exclaimed, "Wallace, there's some calves wandering through my sheets, they'll get them all dirty!" She stood up and reached for her coat. "I'm going out to shoo them away."

Wallace looked out the window. "You'd better not go out there with your broom like you do to Nellie's cow. Those aren't calves; they're Sam's steers, and they can be mean. I'll go over and ask Butch if he'll get the word to him to send in a couple of hired men to round them up."

"And in the meantime they'll wash their backs walking through my wash?" She opened the back door and stood on the stoop, ready to defend her stew and her washing. Not seeming to mind the intrusion, the steers ambled across the yard. Satisfied she'd scared them off, Ethel went back inside.

"As if I didn't have enough to do." Ethel filled the kettles with water and put them on the stove.

While waiting for the water to heat, Ethel thought of Elsie. Writing when new things happened had been a habit for so long, but now she felt different, with a new respect for her daughter and her choices.

> *January 1919*
>
> *My dear Elsie—Happy New Year. I hope you got my letters and cards following your grandparents' death. It sounds like you were a big help to both of them in their illness, and I often wonder whatever they would have done without you. You have had much grief over the last year, and I pray God will comfort you.*
>
> *This is just a quick note to tell you about our wedding. It was a lovely ceremony. I will be sure to send you a picture. Raymond did a very good job of holding my ring, even if he took it away for a few minutes during the service to look at it. I placed your picture on the sideboard so it would be included in the wedding pictures. Everything worked out well. We had some fresh flowers even in December. The bank manager sent roses, and the Sawyers had a poinsettia. They made Christmas special, and Raymond loved our big tree.*
>
> *We're in for another bad winter, I'm afraid. I didn't think anything could be as bad as last year, but so far we have more snow and extremely high winds, and it's been very cold. I've never heard the wind howl as it does here.*
>
> *I'm finally going to write my nurse's registration and really looking forward to doing it. I hope many good things fill this year for you. Always remember that I love you.*
>
> *Wallace and Raymond send their best.*
>
> *Love, Mum*

Ethel put the letter in the envelope and sealed it shut. Wallace could take it to the post office later.

"You want these flowers watered?" Wallace returned unexpectedly, interrupting her thoughts as he came into the room.

She enjoyed her membership in the Edgerton Horticultural Society, and even though she didn't have much time for flowerbeds or a garden, she grew a few vegetables to eat and pampered geraniums through the winter months to later plant in her window boxes.

"I guess the fair is getting better every year, from what the old-timers say," Wallace said. "They tell me the first one in 1911 was out at Challengers. A good one, right from the beginning."

Walking over to her plants, Ethel said with pride, "My plants get better every year too. If these keep up their growth, they should be beauties by spring." There weren't many flowers around the community, and she liked to share what she had.

"It looks like it's going to be a year for babies…1919 began with a bang," Ethel said to Wallace as she sat beside him.

"I guess that's the result of families being reunited after the war," Wallace said.

"The doctor, nurses and all the available helpers are busy," Ethel said. "It doesn't seem to matter if the women live just off Main Street or at the end of a long lane in the country; they look for support of the doctor and willing workers." She picked up her knitting, thinking it'd been so long since she'd knitted that she'd probably forgotten her pattern. "And it's not only babies who need medical care. I think there's more influenza around than what people want to admit. Both those families Doc and I went to see last week were victims."

"House calls aren't the easiest work. You're pretty lucky to have so much help."

"I got some good news this morning. Well, I think it is," Ethel said. "I hear that Lottie's pregnant. You remember her and Ben out the south road. I guess she'd be a couple of months along, and both of them are so happy."

"You'll have your work cut out for you with her!" Wallace grinned and leaned back on his chair.

Later that evening, as Ethel sat at her kitchen table, she thought about her nursing skills and reflected on Doctor Austin's words about working in Canada. Her mind was on the upcoming examination, and she read her nursing books every opportunity she had.

The time soon came for Ethel to make the trip by train into Edmonton to attend the hospital's preparatory classes given to all trained nurses who had applied for their Canadian registration. She accepted Lillian's offer of a winter coat and packed a few personals for the trip.

It was the first time Ethel had returned to Edmonton since she had left almost two years before. Her life had changed so much. How she wished she could go to the cemetery to visit Tom's grave, but there wasn't time. She thought fondly of Mrs. Farrow and their many conversations. She'd be so proud of Ethel's strides of confidence with nursing in the country.

The hospital was familiar to Ethel as she entered through the big wooden doors. She quickly found the classroom and received her instructions for the preparation time. A three-hour examination would follow, and then one of the resident doctors would interview her. She was comfortable with this procedure, having all her papers from the classes she had attended in England, plus her British accreditation.

Already this winter, they'd delivered babies in a cold bedroom where the wind blew through tarpaper siding, in a one-room house behind sheets hanging on a wire, beside a roaring fire, and in a comfortable front bedroom with doors. It was never the same. Her rural experiences in Edgerton were of great value, and she drew from them and the textbooks to answer the questions with confidence.

The classes and examination went well. The interview was challenging, and the discussion stimulating. Ethel eagerly answered the questions. The doctor appeared pleased and encouraged her in her chosen profession. Wishing Ethel well, he shook her hand and said he'd be personally writing a letter.

Ethel returned home feeling confident. She noticed a neighbour's empty pot in her dry sink that had contained either soup or stew. Crumbs from Mrs. Sawyer's freshly baked biscuits lay scattered beside the pot. Family and friends had obviously looked after the family while Ethel was away.

"Wallace, you know what I read in an old newspaper out at the Patterson's house?" Ethel asked one evening after supper. "On October 11th, 1916, Nellie McClung came to speak to the Methodist ladies right here in Edgerton. I guess a lot of people turned out to hear her strong opinions. There was even a charge of fifty cents to hear her. That's pretty steep back then. I wish I had been there."

"You like her, Ethel?"

"I do. My friend in Edmonton, Mrs. Farrow, used to tell me about Nellie McClung and some of her associates. You know, it's women like Nellie who come out to the people and talk to them that open minds and get folks thinking. Maybe she's one of the reasons why people in her circles are fair about many things. I heard her once in Edmonton. She was something. Her words rang true for me."

"I hear she speaks against some behaviour that people accept as normal and important. Some don't like to change their minds, you know," Wallace challenged.

"Like what? Temperance issues? Responsibility to family? Women voting? Thinking? Come on now, Wallace, you and I both know that some of that business should have been swept clean long ago."

"When she gets going about equality," Wallace said, "it raises people's hackles."

Ethel laughed. "So you have been keeping up with her. I left that issue for you to raise."

Even with her teasing, and as tired as she was, she didn't want to admit that her opinion was just that…her opinion. But Wallace would understand.

With her examination behind her, Ethel felt a new surge of energy. Over the next couple of months, she and Wallace painted and wallpapered; he put a new doorframe in the kitchen and fixed the basement steps. All the time they worked, Ethel thought about Tina and Molly Patterson and wondered how they were getting along through the winter.

chapter sixteen

Perfect Timing

Wallace brought in the mail and laid it on the table. Ethel immediately reached for it. There, boldly with black print, was a letter from the University of Alberta. It was Ethel's registration.

There hadn't been a day that Ethel hadn't thought of it. She looked at Wallace, and then she carefully opened the envelope and lifted the stationery from its cover. She didn't want to damage any part of the letter by hurrying.

"Listen, Wallace." Ethel read,

> "We are pleased to inform you that your nursing credentials have been upgraded to Registered Nurse as of this date. Thank you for carrying on the tradition of caring for others."

The enclosed letter listed the various marks for the examinations, the interview and the practical work. She had done exceptionally well.

Ethel cupped her face in her hands. "Isn't that grand? What a load lifted from my shoulders! I feel like dancing."

"I knew you'd pass," Wallace commented as he took her in his arms and waltzed around the room. "I had no doubt in my mind." He planted her squarely on her feet and said, "Don't move." Turning to the cupboard, he stretched to open a drawer, reached to the back and then slowly drew his hand out. Placing a small hard object in her hand, he closed her fingers over it.

"Oh, Wallace," Ethel said. "Is this what I think it is?"

"I hope so." He grinned.

She opened her fingers, looked down at her lapel watch and saw the second hand trip from one mark to another as it circled the small face.

"I thought you'd need this more than ever, now," Wallace said.

"You've given me back many memories with this watch, Wallace." She reached up and hugged him. "Thank you so much."

He opened the fastener on the back of the watch and pinned it on her apron bib. "Now you can nurse me all you want." He laughed aloud.

The news of Ethel's achievement spread around the community; people congratulated her personally and sent their best wishes by mail.

The next week, Ethel decided to go out to the country to visit a couple of families, as well as to tell the good news to Lottie and Ben Mundle. The first families were home and welcomed her with conversation, refreshments and an afternoon of visiting.

Approaching the Mundles' farm lane later that day, Ethel noticed a large red rag tied to Ben's gate. She pulled back on the reins to slow down the horse and turn it into the laneway.

She wondered if Lottie had started her labour and hoped she wasn't too late. After jumping from the buggy, she tied the horse up at the gate. Clutching her small black bag, she rapped loudly on the door and then pushed it open.

"Mrs. Bullymore," Ben said, standing in the kitchen wringing his hands, "am I ever glad you're here. I left a message in town for you or the doctor to come right out."

"Good thinking about the red rag, Ben. How's Lottie?" Ethel went to the stove, poured hot water into a basin and began to wash her hands. Dumping it into the swill pail, she took the green soap out of her bag, poured fresh hot water into the basin and started scrubbing.

"She's doing all right, I guess. I don't really know." Ben grimaced and looked down. "She's early, you know. We were going to have you come out for a few days next week in case she started."

"Well, I'm here now," Ethel said. "Do you think she means business?"

"I really hope so. I know I'm ready. I got a good fire on here. The water's hot on the back of the stove, and Lottie's been baking newspapers, so we have lots of clean sheets to put under her. She's also been boiling cloths, so I got packets of them too. I put a piece of strong rope at the head of the bed and three boards under the mattress like you told me. It should be good 'n straight for her, and there's a rubber sheet and newspapers under the bedsheets. She's ready for you. And, ma'am," Ben said softly, shifting from one foot to another, "Lottie packed a little box of clothes for the baby in case…in case she…she didn't make it."

"Now don't you talk like that, Ben." Ethel put on a clean apron and smiled. "It sounds like you're well prepared. If we're about to make history, we'd better get started."

She left the kitchen and made her way up a wide staircase. At the top, her eyes scanned a brightly lit hall and four doors open to attractively decorated bedrooms. Lottie and Ben had built this house with a dream of filling it with children, and the two of them lived on in the hope of sharing it with another generation.

Ethel heard sobs smothered by sighs as she entered a bedroom. Lottie's eyes squeezed tight in pain while her hands clutched the side of the bed, responding to strong contractions.

"Hello, Lottie," Ethel said softly. "Starting to bring your little one into the world, are you? Good for you."

"Mrs. Bullymore, thanks for coming…oh, I didn't think I'd start this soon…I should have remembered that from my other babies," Lottie said through ragged breaths. "This has gone on too long. But thanks, oh, thank you for being here with me and Ben."

"You're welcome, luv," Ethel said, "so just let baby make its way. I'm here with you, and we're going to have us a little one." Ethel spoke almost in rhythm, acknowledging Lottie's pains.

"I'm afraid, Mrs. Bullymore. I'm just so afraid," Lottie said.

"I know, Lottie, but you're going to be fine. All our talks we've had over the past months are going to work for us now. You just let me do some thinking for you, and you help your body do what it's been made to do. We'll get you all ready to have your baby by the time the doctor gets here."

Several hours passed. Lottie's pains were consistently close together. Ethel was beginning to think that the doctor hadn't gotten Ben's message. Just as she admitted to herself that she was on her own, the doctor burst into the room. "Am I too late for the action?" He winked at Ethel. "Was I ever glad to see your rig in the yard. How're we doing?" He looked down at Lottie. "Having ourselves a baby, are we, Lottie?"

"Oh…Doc, you almost missed it," Lottie panted. "Mrs. Bullymore's got me real close."

"Good. So there's nothing left to do but just catch him?" Turning to Ethel, Doc said softly, "You've got her this far, Ethel; go ahead and finish."

Ethel coached Lottie to push with authority one minute and with a gentle sisterly attitude another.

She glanced at the doctor, and he nodded his consent. After she eased out one shoulder, and then the other, the baby slipped into her hands.

"Oh, Lottie, you did it! It's a boy, and a handsome one at that."

"Is he all right?" Lottie said. "Are you sure he's okay?" Her shoulders shook with sobs.

Ethel held his head down and wiped his mouth clean.

"He's good," she said, directing her attention back to the baby. "Come on, baby, cry," Ethel coaxed. "Come on, baby, you've worked too hard not to breathe this sweet air."

Lottie lifted herself on her elbows to watch. "Oh, please God, give him breath," she cried.

"He'll cry, Lottie," the doctor said. "He'll cry."

Ethel carefully supported the baby's spine while lowering his head. She flicked his feet gently with her fingertips, and the baby gave a couple of gasps, followed by a strong wail. His little face turned pink as he proudly announced his arrival.

"Thank you, baby, well done." Ethel laughed and turned to Lottie. "You did it, Lottie. The baby's beautiful. You're fine. Good for you. It's almost over now."

Tears flooded Lottie's eyes. Ethel could see relief, exhaustion and gratitude across her countenance. An anxious Ben burst into the room and immediately went to Lottie and grasped her hand.

"Ben, you've got yourself a hired hand," the doctor teased him. "A handsome baby, he is. Come look at your son. What would you think, about seven pounds or so? Looks like we were all out on our dates; he looks ready to me."

Ben looked at his son and then turned to Lottie. "How are you, my love? Are you all right?"

"Yes; tired, but I'm so happy. Ben, we've got our young'un after all these years."

Ben put his hands to his head. His shoulders shook in sobs. Quickly wiping his face on the sleeve of his shirt, he looked at the baby again as if in disbelief. "What a difference a moment makes in a man's life. I'm a father again. A bouncer, isn't he?"

After Ethel washed the baby, she wrapped him in a blanket and put him in his mother's arms, soothing him with quiet words. "We'll get you started on nursing."

Ben and Lottie watched their new baby's contented movements.

"We have our baby now, Ben. We're a family."

"Yes, Lottie…thank you. I don't ever want you to go through that again."

"Right now, it's the farthest thing from my mind." She looked at him and smiled. "We've been waiting long enough for him, haven't we, luv? He looks like a Benjamin John, doesn't he?"

Ben stroked Lottie's brow as Ethel closed her eyes and offered a prayer of thanksgiving for God's good gifts and the miracle of new life. Their twilight years would have a bright light in them as they would watch their little boy grow in wisdom and stature.

"Come on, B.J. You've worked hard today," Ethel said. "How'd you like to get some sleep and let your momma rest too?"

Ethel placed B.J. in his basket and walked back to Lottie and Ben. "How do you feel now, Lottie?"

"I'm fine, really. Tired, but so happy." She reached out her hand to Ethel. "When you asked B.J. to let his momma rest, I felt so good. I haven't had anybody to call me Momma for such a long time, and well, what you said sounded so right. Thank you."

"I'm going to ask Isabelle to stay with you and Ben for a while. It'll be a big help to you if she stays for a week. I'm sure she'd like to help you out." Ethel took a step closer to Lottie and said, "Now before I go, I want to make the announcement I came for in the first place before I saw your red flag." She laughed. "I got my results from Edmonton, and I passed with honours."

"Well, congratulations," Doc said, "your first delivery as a R.N. with the one who encouraged you to write the examination. Couldn't have worked that out better."

"I'm so glad for you and not surprised," Lottie said. "As for Isabelle, I was hoping and praying for some help. That'll be perfect. There's cooked meat hanging in the cold room and pies, cookies and muffins on the pantry shelves, along with jams and preserves. Isabelle and Ben won't have any problem finding us something to eat."

News quickly spread of B.J.'s safe arrival. Over the next few weeks, people told Ethel they'd visited Lottie and Ben, taking gifts and food—typical country people, always ready to care for one another.

On a quiet afternoon later that week, Ethel opened her new box of writing stationery to tell Elsie the news.

July 1919

Happy Birthday, Elsie. It's a big one—13. I hope you have a wonderful day. Did you get your card? Thank you for the lovely letter. I enjoy getting news from home so much; it's just like a little visit.

You will be glad to know that I received my nursing registration and I'm very happy about it.

A neighbour brought over two pairs of boots yesterday that were too small for her sons. Guess what? Both pair fit Raymond. So now he has some boots to tromp around in the dirt. And we have lots of that when it rains.

Over the last year, I've helped deliver babies, baked cookies, taken hot meals to neighbours, and nursed everything from the flu to gout. I even set a broken leg for the neighbour's dog. I enjoy my work and the people out here, so much.

This is just a quick letter, so I'll go for now, dear. Say hello to all our family back there.

Wallace, Raymond, and I send our love.

Ethel passionately watched 13-year-old girls like Tina and Isabelle, seeing how they dressed and how they enjoyed each other's company. It was in times like this that she thought about her younger sisters and Elsie.

A Girl's Club had opened in Wainwright, and Ethel read articles in the paper about their meetings. She wanted to learn more about the possibility of having a club in Edgerton. Asking around, she found there were others interested in the club, so she invited two of the Wainwright leaders to meet at her home, along with several girls and their mothers.

One of the leaders came out a few times to get them started. Then Ethel and another interested mother continued. Ethel could not believe this good fortune. She was ecstatic at having all these girls around her. Why hadn't she thought of this sooner? They'd teach her so much about a girl's life in the home, community and school.

She gave Tina and Isabelle some extra responsibilities, and they planned a year of meetings. She thought of some speakers who'd come and talk to the girls, women who could influence them and help them feel valued. She sent out letters and listened for interest among the townspeople. She soon found that people of all ages wanted to contribute money and energy to assist in the formation of the group.

Working at her various interests, there was never enough time for Ethel to spend with Wallace. One night she determined it would be different. She cooked a nice meal and sent Raymond and Isabelle over to the Cozy Café for their supper. She set candles on the table and made Wallace's favourite chocolate cake for dessert.

"What's all this?" he asked as he sat down at the table.

"It's a special night," Ethel answered.

"Oh, yeah? For what?"

"Not for what—but for whom?" Ethel joked.

"Why? We got company coming?" he asked.

"No, just you and me. I thought it'd be nice to have supper together…just us." Ethel set the pot roast on the platter. "I want you to know, Wallace Bullymore, that I appreciate you. You're the love of my life, and I want to say thank you in a special way."

"Well, what do you know about that? I always knew it, but it's nice to hear you admit it." He chuckled.

"You're absolutely right, and I'm going to say it more from now on. I don't ever want to take you for granted," Ethel said. "And there's something else I've been thinking about. You're so good with Raymond, and he loves you. That means a lot to me. You're a man with a big heart, and I love you."

Even as Ethel said that, she knew he'd be asked to share her at any time, but she always wanted to keep him foremost in her mind and heart.

chapter seventeen

Slowing Down

Roy MacGregor, a strong husky lad from north of town, leaned against a tree one afternoon as Wallace and Ethel drove up in their buggy from visiting friends in Ribstone.

"Goodness, I hope Sally and the baby are all right," Ethel said to Wallace. "Sally's baby was premature—it's a miracle he lived."

"Howdy, Mrs. Bullymore, Wallace." After the greetings, Roy turned to Ethel. "Ma'am, awful sorry to bother you, but Sally's got real tired all at once. She don't have much milk to feed the baby. He won't sleep and we can't sleep and, well, I'm a mite worried. I'm wonderin' if you could come out for a spell. I'd drive you, ma'am, if you could spare the time."

Relieved to hear in Roy's remarks that the baby was all right and just having a bit of trouble feeding, Ethel glanced at Wallace. Hidden within his nod was a subtle expression of acceptance.

"Of course, Roy. Let me get a few things and check on some supper for the family. Why don't you go down to the Cozy Café and see if you can find somebody to have a cup of coffee with? Come back for me in an hour."

As Roy and Ethel headed north through town later in the afternoon, she relaxed in the buggy, feeling that everything was fine at home and hoping there was nothing serious with Sally.

"I'm real happy you could come, Mrs. Bullymore."

"I am too, Roy. It's funny how days go by and I never leave the house, and then all at once, I'm never home. We've had a raft of babies this summer. Been pretty busy with them, and then with all the flu cases that seem to be with us again—it keeps us going."

Ethel always enjoyed the north road out of town, down Challenger Hill toward Bloomington Valley. It was a refreshing day, and Roy was good company.

After driving over a sandy knoll and through a grove of trees, they soon pulled up beside a small tarpaper house. Inside, Sally sat in a chair, holding her crying baby. As soon as she saw Ethel, she began to cry too.

"Here, here, Sally. Let me take your baby. What's his name?"

Sally replied through her tears, "Howard, after Roy's father."

"Howard, a good strong name for a bouncing big baby. What is he now, about three months old?"

Sally nodded.

Turning back toward the baby, Ethel touched his cheek. "Howard, you were just about four pounds when I saw you last. It's your momma's good care that's brought you along." Turning toward Sally, Ethel continued, "You've done well with him."

"I couldn't have done it without you, Mrs. Bullymore," Sally said. "I remember the night he was born and the many hours you sat and encouraged me. You knew what to do after he was born, when both him and me was so tired. Doc Smith and you made a good team."

"Ah, we just did what had to be done," Ethel said.

Sally continued, "He would've died if you hadn't been here. I'm sure he would've died. He was so small—such a little baby. After Doc went home, remember how you kept him all warm and comfortable on the oven door? And gave me a time to rest."

Ethel held little Howard close. "For a baby who had a rough start like he did, he's a pretty good size now. Are you able to give him lots of milk?"

"I think I have lots of milk, but even when he's done nursing, he's still hungry."

"Maybe a fine boy like this wants something to chew. Let's fix him a little mush. He's plenty young yet, but he's a big one, and he might need more than milk to satisfy his appetite."

With the baby in one arm and a wooden spoon in the other, Ethel stirred the mush over the open fire. She poured it into a bowl to cool and then began to feed Howard. He opened his mouth, devoured the mush and looked for more.

"You just relax now, Sally. Sometimes a baby this big needs a little extra. He's come along fast from his birth weight. Here now, you bunny him up and nurse him."

Sally cuddled her baby, and in five minutes, he was sound asleep at her breast.

Slowing Down

"What's this about you being so tired?" Ethel asked.

"I just can't get going. I managed to put in a garden, but I'm not able to look after it. I've cut an old coat into enough squares to make a quilt, but I run out of strength before I get them sewn together. Mrs. Bullymore, I just don't have the energy to look after Howard, Roy and the house. It's not like me, ma'am. I love my husband and home. What's the matter with me?"

Ethel looked into her soft violet eyes. "It was a long, difficult winter, Sally. Remember? You had a lengthy confinement, and the birth of your baby was not an easy one. You've probably outdone yourself by putting in your garden and doing housework. Besides, look at all the love and energy you share with Roy and little Howard, doing those extra tasks. With the work and all, it's no wonder you're tired. That's not a problem. It's a natural result."

Looking around the room, Ethel could see where Sally's broom was never still. The furniture, creatively arranged, formed a comfortable setting; the shine on the floors and windows boasted a conscientious housekeeper. "Are these new curtains on the window?"

"Yes," Sally said with pride. "I made them from a couple of sheets and sewed eyelet on them."

"And are those freshly crocheted doilies?"

"Yes, I just starched them. I found some cotton ones in a box that belonged to Howard's mother."

Ethel picked up a newly crocheted afghan. "My dear Sally." Ethel smiled. "I want you to slow down and enjoy your baby and husband. The good Lord will look after growing the garden, and the housework can wait. You need to take care. Spoil yourself. Be good to Sally." Ethel took the edge of the afghan and placed it around Sally's shoulder and then tucked the bottom under the baby.

"Try to keep your milk for another three months. During that time, you'll gather strength to take in the garden as it ripens. Don't forget you've got to make meals for the harvesters soon. Drink lots of juices, make sure you get eight hours sleep every night and enjoy an afternoon nap while Howard has his."

Sally laughed. "I know you're right. I've been working hard. I promise to change."

Ethel turned as Roy came in from the barn. "I should be getting along." With a wink she added, "Everything's fine here. Sally's doing a good job. A nice boy you've got there, Roy."

With one last look at little Howard, Ethel made her way to the door.

chapter eighteen

Different-sized Gifts

The fall passed slowly, and the population of Edgerton increased. Ethel teased the mothers about rushing to deliver before another hard winter set in. She and Doc had been out to many farmhouses, giving folks early Christmas presents. Little children had been thrilled to see a cradle under their tree.

The town transformed into a fairyland with candles burning in the windows. Red bows hung on doorframes and railings as Christmas drew closer. Ethel loved this time of year. She began to think about her first wedding anniversary and community events in the festive season. One of the annual highlights was the South District school's Christmas concert.

Ethel sat at the kitchen table colouring a poster to put up at the grocery store as a last minute reminder. A sharp knock interrupted her thoughts. She opened the door to find the youngest member of the South District School Board.

"Hello, Mrs. Bullymore," he said. "I'm glad you're home. I need to talk to you. It's about the concert this afternoon. We won't be needing your cookies."

"What are you telling me?" Ethel asked. She straightened to her full height to confront her visitor.

"I'm…I'm just sayin', ma'am, that we're cancelling the concert. My pa's always been Santa, and he's been in bed for two weeks with his arthritis. And besides, he says there's a storm blowin' up from the east that'll give us bad roads. The teacher didn't want to cancel, but it looks like there's no other choice."

Ethel stood on her front porch facing him, not extending an invitation to come any further, in spite of the brisk wind. "Of course there's another choice. Don't cancel," she said. "The children have been looking forward to this concert for a month, and it's their last day of school before Christmas. Do you realize how much memory work they've learned? Come on now, you remember what it was like when you were a kid. The Christmas concert was the highlight of the year. It still is."

"I'm real sorry, ma'am, but Pa is just too sick, and the parents probably won't come if it's stormy."

"Now, truthfully, is it the fact that your father has never missed being Santa or is it the storm? I'm sorry he's ill. I'll go to see him myself, if that'll help." She turned towards the front hall, lifting her hand to invite the young man to enter the house. "This concert must not be cancelled. We can get another Santa—no offence to your father. The storm, well, if it comes, we can't do much about that. I know you came to tell me not to bother bringing the cookies for the lunch, but I'll just take them and give them to the children. Maybe they can have a concert, big or small, Santa or no Santa—good roads or bad." She smiled at the young man, hoping she hadn't offended him. "Maybe I'll be the only one to applaud."

"How're you going to tell them there won't be a Santa?" The young man pleaded as he wrung his hands and paced up and down the hallway. "Children are used to singing 'Jingle Bells' and seeing Santa run down the aisle ringing his bell. What kind of ending can you possibly give to the concert that'll compare with a jolly old Santa?"

"Never mind, young man; you just let people bring their cookies and leave the rest up to me," Ethel said.

"But ma'am, I think you're making a big mistake. They need a Santa, and they need parents there to watch them give their lines. They look forward to doing their bowing and curtsying and hearing people applaud."

"Don't tell the parents this." Ethel chuckled. "But half the fun of the concert is for the children to perform the work they practiced. Sure, it's nice to have their parents, and if the storm doesn't come, well, I'm sure they'll be there. But at least the children will get a chance to say their lines. And, yes, Santa will visit and give them candy canes." Ethel shrugged and lowered her voice. "I don't know how, yet, but I don't want those children disappointed. It wouldn't be fair if we cancelled."

By noon, clouds had spread across the sky, hiding it from view, indicating the inevitable storm. The wind blew, and the heavy air cushioned the snowflakes as they fell and formed snowbanks along the ditches and across the roads. Ethel watched out the window and hoped she'd made the right decision.

The concert began as expected with quite a few parents present. Verse after verse of accurately spoken memory work reflected the dedication of teacher and

Different-sized Gifts

child, as well as their appreciation of literature. The playlets, performed with humour and precision, pleased the small audience. Ethel arranged the cookies and fruitcake on a side table and set out cups.

When the master of ceremonies came to the end of the program, he appeared uncertain as to what he should say. He looked around at everyone and rubbed his mouth with the back of his hand. Ethel hoped he wouldn't say "This is the end of the program" with 15 pairs of eyes looking at him and expecting him to announce Santa Claus.

He cleared his throat and ran his fingers through his hair, looked down at the children and took a deep breath. "Maybe we should sing a couple of Christmas carols." Instantly, the music of "Hark the Herald Angels Sing" filled the room.

When the last verse was almost over, a loud outburst of bells followed by a hearty "Ho, ho, ho," got people's attention. The children laughed and jumped up and down in their seats. The teacher immediately began to play "Jingle Bells," and everyone joined in as Santa bounced into the room. The parents applauded, and a man put his fingers to his lips and whistled loudly.

One by one, the children sat on Santa's knee and disclosed their secret wishes. Santa gave them a candy cane, told them to be good boys and girls and, after a hug, lifted them down. Excited, they darted to their seats, eager to watch Santa talk to their friends.

During the chorus "For He's a Jolly Good Fellow," Santa ran to the back, tucking a large, rather bulky stomach in behind the big black belt, laughing and shouting a hearty "Merry Christmas to all, and to all a good night!" Striking the chords for a carol, the teachers led the parents in more singing.

Just as Ethel slipped into the back row during the last verse, one of the trustees said, "Were you helping Santa on his way, Mrs. Bullymore?"

"Indeed, I was, Charlie. He's busy this time of year."

A rather stunned school board chairman came to the front of the classroom and shook his head. "Well, Santa visited us after all. Come on, folks, the coffee's on the stove, and we have some lunch waiting for us. I'm sorry more parents weren't able to attend this afternoon. Pass the word and tell them what a great concert it was, and a heartfelt thanks to you for braving the weather."

Later that week, the young trustee met Ethel in the grocery store. "Sure was a good concert," he said.

"I'm so glad everything went well. I knew the children would do just fine," Ethel said.

"Can't figure it out though, ma'am. Since you thought it was so all-fired important for the concert to go on, I wondered why you had to leave early. But I'm glad you brought your cookies; I had three of 'em."

"And you enjoyed your trip up to Santa for a candy cane?"

"Ah, Mrs. Bullymore, I guess I'm a big kid at heart. I wanted that concert to go on, really I did. I didn't want to cancel. It just seemed the best thing to do at the time. What with Pa being sick and the roads promising to be bad, I didn't think we had no other choice." He paused, frowned and rubbed his chin. "Hey, how do you know I went up for a candy cane? I mean, who told you? You weren't even there when Santa came."

All at once, he began to laugh, "Or were you, Mrs. Bullymore? Well, I'll be darned if you weren't. Someone told me that maybe you was that Santa, but I had it figured that it was Mr. Bonner. Well, I never."

"I've been stranger things." Ethel headed toward the counter. "Better finish my order."

While Ethel waited for Muriel to add up her groceries, she noticed some folks come in the door and recognized them as a new family in town.

"Tell me something," Ethel asked Muriel. "How are the new folks getting along? Do they have enough money to buy what they want?"

"I don't like to say anything, Mrs. Bullymore," Muriel replied, "but since it's you who's asking, I've noticed they look at something an awful long time before they either decide to buy it or leave it on the counter."

"Do you think they could use a little help, you know, 'til their restaurant business gets better?"

"I don't know if they'd accept help. But if you can think of some way, I have a feeling it'd be like a gift from heaven. I know the missus is a good seamstress, if that's any help. I hear she sewed their winter coats."

Ethel smiled and nodded. She had just the right solution. It would have to be something that wouldn't offend them. Being new, they might not understand this community's generosity. "Thanks, Muriel. Have a nice Christmas," she said, as she left the store.

If she could send Wallace over with a bag and say that somebody had left it at our house for them, giving a gift to the family would be easy. Well, it was true…in a round about way.

That was it. That was exactly what would work. She'd go along in case the missus didn't believe him. *Now what kinds of things can I put in the bag?*

Knowing there were several children in the family helped her decide. She wrapped some mints and chocolates, along with four Christmas bells. Buttons, all sizes and colours, thread and needles, yarn and some knitting needles were carefully added to the pile. Maybe some patches, ribbon, and a new pair of scissors would be helpful, along with a couple of those popular zippers. Ethel had some new material she'd been saving for curtains, but it'd make a nice dress or tablecloth.

She prepared the bag with the mints and bells on top and called Wallace into the room to inform him of her plan. "Just tell her that somebody wants you to give her this bag. I'll explain to her later, if I have to. I'll come, and if she doesn't take it from you, then I'll step up to the door. Isabelle can watch Raymond."

Ethel's peculiar request didn't seem to surprise Wallace. Shrugging his shoulders, he picked up the bag. Together they walked across the street.

After tramping up the outside wooden staircase, he tapped the snow off his boots and knocked on the door. Ethel stood in the shadows at the bottom of the stairs. Following a noisy commotion, a small, dark-haired woman abruptly opened the door and stood looking at him. Several young children, bright eyed with looks of astonishment, tilted their faces to stare up at Wallace. Ethel grinned as she watched from her privileged position.

"Yes, can I help you?" said the young woman. In her anxiety, a pronounced accent tumbled through the strange mix of words.

Wallace said, "I think so, ma'am. My name is Wallace Bullymore. I believe this bag is for you. Someone wants you to have it, and they left it with me to give to you."

"Someone gave it to you…to give to me?" she asked. "How could that be?"

"Can't say for sure, but if it's all right with you, I'll just leave it here."

"No. No. Please do not do that. It cannot be ours. Who would do that? We do not know anybody in town." She put her hands out in front of her body to keep Wallace and his bag at arm's length, as if he held dynamite.

"Believe me, ma'am, stranger things have happened at my house. This is yours. I know it is, so Merry Christmas." He turned to leave.

"No, no, please," she repeated, rejecting the bag.

Ethel thought he was losing the argument until he said with firmness, "Look, it's a gift. Someone gave it to you. It's for you. I'm just the delivery boy, and that's the truth. Now, it's Christmas-time, and you're new, and this is a friendly town. So why don't you just take the bag and keep peace in my family. It's too cold a night to stand in your doorway. Wish me a Merry Christmas and I'll be on my way…please?"

Reluctantly, she reached out her hand, took the parcel from Wallace's arm and offered him a hesitant smile. "Thank you, sir. So, Mrs. Bullymore is your wife?"

"Why, yes, but what does that have to do with it?"

"I will take it and ask no more questions." She chuckled as she slowly turned and closed the door behind her.

Excitement filled the Bullymore household through January. Ethel and Wallace were both very thrilled about expecting a baby in June. She was 36, he was 39, and she knew this would probably be their only child together. Not able to keep their secret, she wrote to Elsie. Ethel thought about the experience of childbirth and looked forward to it once again. With a local midwife-nurse, she'd be able to deliver at home.

Wallace brought in the mail and pleasantly interrupted her several weeks later. A letter from Elsie lay on the top.

> *February 1920*
> *Dear Mummy,*
> *I am so happy to hear of your new baby, and I wonder if Raymond is terribly excited about this. Do take care of yourself and don't work too hard out in the country. The neighbours will want to help you after the care you've given them over the years.*
>
> *I'm glad you went ahead with your nursing examination because I know nursing is important to you.*
>
> *I entered one of my drawings in the winter fair, and I won a prize. I think everybody got something, but I was happy to be mentioned. They put the picture on the class wall.*
>
> *Write to me soon, and tell me how you are feeling.*
> *Your loving daughter, Elsie*

"It's always so good to hear from Elsie."

"It's the next best thing to having her here with us, isn't it?" Wallace said.

"It is, and so important. I take her suggestion not to work too hard very seriously. Over the next while, I think I'll only take nursing calls in town; there are others who can go out to the country."

chapter nineteen

The Town Gathers

Days turned into weeks as Ethel looked forward to spring. The sun shone warmly through the windowpane, covering the seeds Ethel had planted in a hotbed.

Life picked up a new pace as spring offered the usual seasonal work. Good weather gave needed rain and ample sunshine, and Ethel saw farmers getting on the land early. People around town talked about the possibility of enlarging the South School District, which was good news, because Ethel knew many young people in the area needed education and the existing schools were overflowing.

A barn-raising had been a big event; the neighbours had worked hard to help a local rancher prepare for the expected harvest.

And tonight was the annual garden party on Sandersons' yard. "We'll need to be down there by four o'clock to help set up tables," Ethel told Wallace.

When Ethel's list was complete, she and Wallace packed their baskets and walked down the street. When the time came to eat, the music stopped and people gathered in lines beside the large tables in the backyard to fill their plates from an abundant variety of food. Coal oil lanterns hung from the poles, lighting up the white picket fence and spacious lawn. Spring flowers, tiger lilies and fireweed bouquets graced the tables.

Suddenly, a deep voice resonated through the night air, and a few people shushed those who were talking.

"Let's give thanks. God of bountiful love and good gifts, we thank you for pouring your grace on us. Thank you for helping us to be a community and care for one another. Bless this place, this food, and us to your service. Amen."

Following the hum of amens across the people, Rev. Taylor, the Methodist minister, gave the invitation for the folks to pick up a plate and move forward. Ethel looked over the table where local farmers had brought barbecued meat.

"Quite a spread, Wallace," Ethel said. "Nobody's going to go home hungry."

Spoons and forks stood in pots of hot potatoes, sliced carrots, shredded cabbage, turnip and stewed tomatoes.

"Not to mention the dessert table," Wallace said as he looked over the tarts, cakes and sweet-lemon pies.

"It'll take you a while to get through all of this." Ethel glanced at chokecherry jam spilled over the edges of freshly baked muffins, proving the baking skills of the women of Edgerton and district.

Following the meal, and after an evening of visiting and toe-tapping music, Ethel and Wallace gathered their empty plates and dishes and trudged home with a tired Raymond.

The Bullymore household settled quickly as a long day and fun-filled evening ended. A mantle of silk-like dark clouds covered the sky, shutting out the stars and giving the night a peaceful disguise. Gentle winds brushed against the windowpanes, contributing to the rhythm of ongoing sleep.

Suddenly, a pounding on the front door echoed as if an army had marched across the veranda. The dog barked, and Wallace's feet hit the floor with a thud. Raymond cried out, and Ethel ran to look through the window but couldn't see anything. Not even a horse or rig tied to the rail.

She hurried down the stairs and pulled the door curtain aside to see the framed faces of Margaret Lehman and Butch Bonner. Quickly, she opened the door.

"Evenin', Ethel. Sorry to wake you up, but Margaret here…well, she needs your help. The missus has the children. We didn't want her to go home from the party feeling like she is."

"Come in, Margaret. Thanks, Butch, I appreciate you bringing her."

One look at Margaret and Ethel knew there was no time to waste. She'd noticed her at Sandersons' earlier and thought she'd be delivering this baby soon. After calling up the staircase for Wallace to go fetch the doctor, and to hurry, Ethel guided her into the front bedroom. She made her comfortable and then went to the kitchen to put water on to boil.

Within the half hour, Margaret delivered a big baby boy.

"Mrs. Bullymore did a great job," Margaret said later to the doctor. "She's pretty important to me, and, well…she's been at the birth of all my children. I never knew my mother, and sometimes I secretly think of her that way." Turning to Ethel, she added, "I hope you don't mind."

"Margaret, my dear, I don't mind a bit, but I'll tell you a secret." Ethel patted her shoulder, winked at her and whispered, "I don't want to be at the birth of another child next year." With a little humour in her voice she continued, "You tell your man you need breathing space." Ethel paused, choosing her words carefully. "Three children in three years is enough. There's more to life than having babies. You need time to enjoy them."

Margaret turned her head, looked out the window and smiled. Ethel could see she liked what she'd heard, but she had probably never allowed herself to think so boldly.

"I'll go now, "Doc Smith said, "and leave you in Ethel's capable hands.

"Thank you for coming, Doctor."

Margaret turned to Ethel. "I needed to hear that. You know, what you said about more to life than having babies. I keep thinkin' another baby might bring Burt and me closer together."

"That's the wrong reason for having babies, Margaret. It doesn't work that way."

"I just don't know how I'm going to manage. Heaven knows where he is tonight. Still out there fighting that flaming war in his own way."

"Yes," Ethel replied softly, "heaven knows." Six months after he'd gone to war, Burt had physically come home, but emotionally he was still there. "The war took the heart out of many a good man. May God be with him, wherever he is."

"Mrs. Bullymore, if God has angels of mercy down here on earth, you're sure to be one of them."

"I'm sure God has, and thanks for that lovely thought. You have a nap. I'm going to my room for a little rest before the day begins."

Ethel lay on her bed and thought about Margaret and her man. Sometimes life didn't seem too kind to folks.

Following considerable time, she dressed and went into the kitchen to prepare breakfast. After putting together an attractive tray for Margaret, she carried it into the front bedroom.

"Good morning. Did you get some sleep?" Ethel asked.

"I did. And this little one makes me forget all about the pain." The baby squirmed in his blanket and sucked his fists. When Margaret looked up, Ethel was surprised to see her face streaked in tears.

"I…I've been doing a lot of thinking. I don't know how I'm going to raise another child. Maybe…maybe I should give them up." Margaret sobbed.

Ethel took a deep breath and moved to the edge of her chair.

"I don't think so, Margaret. The good Lord didn't give you these children so you could give them away to someone else. You are to provide for them the best you can and raise them to be good citizens, just like you are. But there are no rules about how you provide for and raise them. They can eat vegetables from my garden; they can wear hand-me-downs. That never hurt anybody. And when the cold nights start, they can keep warm from wood brought from somebody else's bush. We just need to make some arrangements. We'll get this organized. People need people, Margaret; there's nothing wrong with that. Right now, you need us, and we're going to help you. The children belong with their mother, and I for one am not going to stand by and see them lose her."

"Oh, Mrs. Bullymore." Margaret reached over to the side table for her handkerchief. "I'm easily talked out of it. I feel so guilty every time I think of giving them up. Then I feel so guilty for keeping them when I can't look after them the way I should."

"Margaret, I know what you mean, but there are different ways to work this out. My mother offered to help me with my daughter for 10 years because of circumstances beyond my control. But I never gave her away, even though I couldn't raise her." Ethel looked directly at her, cleared her throat and wiped her brow. Very slowly she continued, "Your man now, he's a different story, but that doesn't make you any less a parent. I know you love your children, and that's what's important."

"Thank you, ma'am."

"Don't worry, luv. We'll find a way." Ethel gave her a hug and then turned, picked up the soiled baby laundry and walked towards the washtub. *God help me. Between us, we can do this.*

chapter twenty

Celebration in the Midst of Life

Wallace pulled a chair out for Ethel to sit down at the breakfast table.

"To what do I credit such formality this morning?" she said. "Afraid I'll burn your toast?"

"Nope, just thought I'd start the day off in a pleasing way," Wallace said.

Sitting down beside her, he picked up the *Chauvin Chronicle* and began to glance across the headlines. "Some interesting activities going on at the church, I see."

Ethel enjoyed her membership in the Anglican congregation and hoped in the near future that they'd have their own church building, rather than sharing premises with the Methodists as they were doing at this time. She mixed with the people in worship and fellowship at a different level than through her nursing. She asked advice on issues around the town and learned about their faith as she spent time with them.

"We can't complain about being bored. I guess that's a good thing about a small town. People get things going, and soon they've got an organization, or a building, or some group all fired up." Wallace took a bite of his toast and flipped the rest to his dog. "Sure can't get any games better than curling, hockey and baseball."

"Aw, with your competitive spirit, you don't miss an opportunity to plug sports. If one of those games is going on," Ethel said, and then she laughed as she wiped her hands on the dish towel, "you're going to be there, either cheering or playing."

Ethel looked at the back of the page that Wallace held. "Soon going to need more room to tell all the news."

"I hear there's a benefit dance over at Gorton's Hall on Saturday night. Apparently a bunch of the farmers out in the South District got together to see how they could help Molly Patterson. Some of them came up with this idea to give her some cash."

"Why, that's splendid!" Ethel's heart was bursting with pride.

Wallace told Ethel about the progress on the Patterson farm. She was amused because that meant it had been the local talk, and that's how people got help.

Town and farm people would fill Gorton's Hall, a large two-storey building where the community attended concerts, entertainment and dances. If they got tired of the two-step, they could always go to another area for a game of pool or cards. But on Saturday night, people would gather around Tina and Molly Patterson with good food, fine music and supportive handshakes. What better medicine is there than friends showing support?

On Sunday morning, dark clouds hung heavily in the sky, and rain threatened. Ethel pulled the bedroom curtains back and clipped them in the window hook. Good feelings remained from the events of the previous night, and it seemed that it'd take more than rain to dampen the spirit of this day.

All the churches united for an outdoor worship service once a year to support one another in the faith and to remind new folks coming to the area about the importance of a church community. People dropped denominational labels, and those who had joined different churches in marriage would sit together as one family.

"Now, if the wind would just blow those storm clouds away, we'd be all set," Wallace said as he carried planks from the wagon to build the seats.

"Maybe it should just rain and get it over with," Herbie, one of the farm men from south of town, added.

"Not a chance. That sky is calling for an all-day rain if I ever saw one," Butch said.

"Well, we're going to keep working anyway," Rev. Taylor said, "and if we have to run for cover, well, that's what we'll have to do. Some people have probably been praying for rain for that dry land south of town, and some people have been praying for sunshine for our service. I suspect God will smile either way." He laughed and picked up a board.

A large crowd gathered at eleven o'clock with black clouds rolling around overhead and thunder rumbling in the distance. Ethel kept holding up the palm of her hand to feel for rain.

Rev. Taylor opened the service and welcomed visitors into the larger faith

Celebration in the Midst of Life

family. His voice resonated deeply through the morning air as he preached and prayed. A community choir, solos and congregational singing offered a grand selection of music.

The minister finished the service by asking the group to celebrate being family as the townspeople of Edgerton: those with faith, those without faith, some with answers, some without even the questions.

With these thoughts resonating in Ethel's mind, she moved out of the crowd and joined the other women who had organized the potluck lunch and had begun to put it on the table.

On the morning of June 20th, Ethel got up very early after having cramps all night and immediately knew they should begin preparations for the home birth. Wallace and Raymond stayed out of the way, but close enough not to miss some of the excitement. When it came time to deliver, Nurse Sturgis attended Ethel and lived up to her reputation of excellence. She put Ethel through her paces so thoroughly and confidently that Ethel thought she was back in London with Nurse Rankin. The doctor was gracious, waiting to go in at the last minute. Ethel gave birth to a boy, and an overwhelming peace filled her as once again she held a baby of her own.

"Let's call him Gordon," Wallace said.

"I like the name very much," Ethel replied. "I'm so thankful it's all over and I have him here in my arms."

"I am too, luv," Wallace said. "Raymond seems excited with having a little brother."

"I'm going to write Elsie and tell her she has another little brother," Ethel said.

"And I'll put that big wooden board on the front veranda and announce the new arrival to the town."

Ethel watched as he got a paintbrush and some brown paint and drew *"It's a Boy. Mum and him doing splendid."*

chapter twenty-one

Ethel's Surprise

Having a baby in the house brought the repetitious task of washing diapers, nursing schedules and sleepless nights. Ethel was determined to do as much as she could herself, but that didn't last long. Thankful for Isabelle's help with the housework and her gift of persuasion, Ethel realized she needed time to rest. Goodness, if she didn't write some of the things down that had happened in the past, she'd never believe them. She began to think about different situations where she'd been involved by helping others.

She opened her journal and wrote,

> I've met so many people in Edgerton that have filled my life with meaning. They have gone out of their way to help me feel at home among them. It's a wonderful community to bring up a family and carve out a life.

Words spilled onto the page so fast, Ethel could hardly write fast enough. She grew excited as the stories took shape in her mind. Yes, this would be an important keepsake of good memories. There were so many accounts to tell. How would she manage to do them justice? She'd just have to write them down as she remembered them and maybe add to them over time. She'd think about where to begin and what to include.

The long period without going out to nurse in the community grew tiresome for Ethel, and she began to attempt small tasks. When Gordon was six weeks old, she took him for his first pram ride, with Raymond helping to push it along the sandy path. They went to the grocery store for some milk and walked into an ongoing dispute.

"Licorice! Licorice! It's mine. Tell them, Mrs. Bullymore, it's mine," children cried as they gathered around her and tugged at her skirt, obliging her to referee their argument.

Ethel listened to the deafening sound of boys arguing while Muriel attempted to solve the problem by opening a new box of licorice.

"Come now, children, enough of this." Kneeling beside them, Ethel gave them each a penny. "Go and get your stick of licorice," she said, raising her voice as the children ran up to the long counter. "Raymond, here's one for you, too."

She wished she could send the children off to someone's yard to play on a swing—they didn't really have a playground of their own. Goodness knows, the adults made sure *they* had enough places. Creating a children's sandbox would be an easy job in this town, with all the sand Edgerton provided underfoot. They'd just have to dig a hole, pick a few stones and build a wooden frame. She'd speak to the reeve in the morning about a park and to Mr. Milne at the lumberyard about the cost of lumber for swings and a teeter-totter and of course a fence.

After settling that in her mind, she paid for her groceries and quickened her steps towards home.

Isabelle had helped Ethel prepare her favourite supper, and it was slowly cooking in the oven of the wood stove. The heat from the stove felt good, as it was cool in the house today.

Roast beef and several kinds of vegetables—she couldn't imagine a nicer meal than that. It was at times like this that she wanted to invite the whole town in to sit down.

"Why not have the Sawyers over and ask Isabelle to help you cook?" Wallace had asked her last week. "It's about that time, isn't it?" *That time* described the yearly tradition after their wedding at Jim Sawyer's house when they'd eaten a wedding dinner together.

"I've been thinking about that, but we don't usually do that until closer to Christmas. I guess it wouldn't matter, though. In fact, we can have them over now and then do it again later." So she prepared for their visit. It had been a long time since she'd entertained, and Ethel looked forward to seeing her old friends around her table.

Now, the day had come, and the last-minute preparations were complete. She walked into the house, placed Gordon in his bassinet, settled Raymond with some building blocks and then noticed several paper bags lying on the side table.

Ethel's Surprise

Placing some items down in the cold room, she saw two cut-glass bowls attractively filled with jellied salads. A large container of vinegar coleslaw sat on the top shelf.

Back in the kitchen, she looked around more closely. After lifting a cloth away from a tray of homemade buns, she observed two loaves of freshly baked bread. Now that she had taken all her groceries off the table and put them away, she also noticed salt and pepper shakers plus sugar and spoons set in the middle on her new turnabout, on a fresh tablecloth.

"This is getting funnier all the time," she said. Noticing the door to the dining room was open, she walked toward it.

"I can't believe this!" she said. Her Sunday cutlery and dishes were all in place on her best linen. Between the two tables, she suspected about 12 to 15 people were coming to supper.

I wish somebody had invited me to my own house. Who would do all this, and who is coming? Where is Wallace, anyway? How can my little blade of beef possibly feed all these people—whoever they are? What are they expecting, another loaves and fishes miracle?

Ethel didn't often feel left out of plans. Usually, she was the one in the centre doing all the arranging, but today she felt excluded. At five o'clock the roast would come out, and it was a quarter to the hour now. She considered what she'd do. First, she needed to freshen up. She changed from her wrinkled housedress to a new cotton dress and combed her dark-brown hair into a tight bun. She applied a little rouge to her cheeks and lips. After pulling on her new oxford shoes, she went back out to the kitchen.

Yes, the roast looked perfect, but she'd have to take it out or it'd turn into leather. Pleased, she put it on a platter, arranged the potatoes and vegetables around its edge and set it up in the warming oven of the big cookstove.

She sat down in the front room and thought about how either somebody had a warped sense of humour or she was losing her ability to remember what this evening was supposed to be. She was not amused.

The hum first sounded like bees gathering around their favourite rosebush. It grew louder and heightened in rhythm from the back part of the house. *What is that irritating noise anyway?* Exasperated, she tucked her apron around her waist, then turned and walked directly into a dozen friends. They immediately broke out in a "Happy Birthday" song. Wallace, the Sawyers, the Bonners and many other friends, dishes in hand, filled her kitchen and overflowed onto the back porch.

"But, we were going to…this was supposed to be—"

"We missed your birthday." Jim Sawyer lifted his hand in response. "And we all decided to catch you when you were sure to be home with your feet up, so here we are. Aren't you going to invite us in?"

Wallace stood beside Ethel, and she grinned up at him. What a grand thing to do! She'd remember this always. They sang "Happy Birthday" again and lit the white candles on the two-tier chocolate birthday cake. "Make a wish and then blow, Ethel," Doc Smith called from the back of the group.

"My wish is for good people like you to continue filling my life. My thanksgiving is being in a town where people care for one another, as you do for my family and me," she responded.

She blew out the candles as everyone sang "For She's a Jolly Good Fellow." Wallace escorted Ethel to the head of the table, bowed graciously and asked her to be seated.

"We have this all planned out now, Ethel. You just relax. Do you mind if we use your roast? I mean, since you went to all the trouble of cooking it?" Everyone laughed. Roast beef was her favourite meal, so they placed two more plates of sliced meat beside hers.

"Let this meal be an opportunity to return to Ethel some of the kindness she so graciously extends to the rest of us." Jim lifted his glass, inviting others to do the same.

"Here! Here!" the group echoed.

"I'm especially going to enjoy this meal," Ethel said. "I've been putting my feet up lately and really slacking off. You're all going to spoil me."

"Aw, but we never know what's around the corner," Eunice said. "In another few months you'll likely be worked off your feet again. So you'd better enjoy this while you can."

On a September afternoon, Ethel laid the newspaper on the table so she could see it better. "Wasn't it nice that Raymond received that award at the Edgerton school fair? He's so proud to see his name printed in the *Chauvin Chronicle*."

"He's famous." Wallace laughed and leaned over to see the article. "The first year they hold the fair, and Raymond is one of the winners! And he really took to hanging the ribbon up so everybody can see it when they come in. That's good. I'm happy for him. It shows he likes to achieve."

"It says here in the paper: 'The exhibits were of splendid quality. Their numbers adequately testified to the interest of both children and parents.' And there was good competition too; Jean Millard, Edith Rusnell and E. Perkins." Ethel folded the newspaper after she read it, content that even Raymond had begun to contribute to the community.

"He's doing well, isn't he, Wallace? I mean, he's adjusted so well to our family life. It's like he doesn't remember all the grief before Edgerton."

"As long as he's happy, Ethel, you can be his memory for him when he needs it."

chapter twenty-two

Double Delights

Winter made an early appearance. Doc had decided to drive today, so Ethel pulled mitts, hats and scarves from their storage; calls to the country caused extra care when driving in cold weather.

The horse trailed through the freshly fallen snow as the sleigh skis sliced the white banks like sharp knives, leaving definite lines across the blanketed area.

"Ethel, I'm feeling a little uneasy about Marie Flander and wondering if we shouldn't go back. Her ankles are swollen and quite dark in colour, and she says that the tips of her fingers are a little numb. She had a bad experience during her last delivery with a doctor who had no regard for her. It's left her a bit shaken for this delivery. What do you think?"

"Yes, we should go back. If we carry on, we'll just worry."

"Then I'll turn around at the next yard. I'd like to bring her into town where we can watch her closely. It's got to be so hard to wait out a difficult labour at the end of a farm lane in the dead of winter."

As Doc reined the horse to the right, the sleigh turned, and they headed back to Flanders' house. His last statement resonated in Ethel's mind. Was this the right time to share her dream of having a maternity home?

"Doc, I've been thinking for some time about turning a room in our house into a nursing area. What do you think of that idea?"

"Great idea, Ethel! Who do you see using it?"

"Well, expectant mothers, anybody who needs care after an accident, anyone who needs you, me or somebody else close to them. It worked well for Margaret Lehman and others who've had their babies there. Other nurses in the area have similar facilities, and in time I'd like to try maternity bed privileges. You know, licensed with the province. Wallace could make some structural changes, and it'd be a good place for women to come. It could be a lying-in and delivering place. And some day I might have a clinic or a private hospital there."

"It sounds good to me. Would Wallace agree to this?"

"I haven't talked it over with him yet. But one good part about it, he'd have me home more."

Doc laughed and drew his reins in tighter to hold the horse back. "I'm sure your home has been a haven to anybody who's been there. Why don't you and Wallace work it out, and if he agrees, then we'll do some planning about supplies and equipment. You'll have to check the government requirements. There'll be regulations and a license to pursue."

"I'd expect that. I'll attend to it as soon as I can."

They came to Flanders' lane and drove up to the neat white dwelling. Smoke poured out of the chimney, inviting them into the warm house. Sam opened the kitchen door for them.

"Thought we'd come back, Sam, before we headed into town."

"Sure glad you did, Doc. Maw started to get some bad stomach cramps and back pains about a half hour ago. What does that mean?"

"Well," Doc said slowly, "it could mean she's going into labour. Then again, it could be that sauerkraut we had for lunch."

Sam smiled, but a frown lay across his worried brow. "Whatever it is, Doc, my worryin' is gettin' the best of me."

Ethel ruffled the hair of the two Flander boys, who stood looking at her. "Are you two scallywags getting ready for a new sister or brother?"

"Yes, ma'am, we're ready. Is our maw ready?" one of the boys asked.

"I don't know. Let's go and see, Doc," Ethel said.

After his usual greeting to Mrs. Flander, Doc examined her, consulted with Ethel and asked Sam to come into the room. "Taking into account the cramps and pain she's had in the last hour, I think you'd better start the water boiling."

Within the hour, Mrs. Flander had made progress. Turning to Ethel, Doc said, "She might need a little help with the pain. The bottle is over there on the table. Moisten that cloth and let her breathe a whiff. I think she's going to require some support with this one."

Ethel hoped the chloroform would relax her so she could finish quickly, as she was tiring.

After a little more coaching, a small pink baby girl slipped from her mother's body. The doctor caught her, flipped her over in a professional grip, cleansed her mouth of mucus and coaxed her to test her vocal cords. The baby cried loudly, and Doc passed her to Ethel. Continuing to give Mrs. Flander his full attention, he said, "Ethel, I do declare, come here. What do you think of this?"

Ethel came around to the end of the bed. "Looks like we've got ourselves another baby."

"You're right. Here comes a contraction. Mrs. Flander, you're not through yet. Come on, push again. What do you think about that, eh? One for each of you."

In a few minutes, another little girl slid from her warm secluded place into the doctor's hands.

He completed the delivery and assured Mrs. Flander that she had two healthy babies. Ethel cleaned up the bed, prepared both babies and then passed them to their mother.

She went into the kitchen to find Mr. Flander and the children waiting anxiously. "Have I got a surprise for you! Mrs. Flander delivered a beautiful baby girl, and then a few minutes later, guess what? She delivered another one. Now, you can't ask for better Christmas presents than that."

Mr. Flander swept the tears away from his eyes. "Well, what do you know? Is she all right…Maw, I mean?"

"She's just fine. She'd like very much for you to come and see the little ones."

The group filed excitedly into the bedroom. Their anticipation, mixed with reverence for this special moment, showed across their countenances.

Sam Flander was the first one to speak. "What do you think, Maw, about having two babies?"

"Very special, indeed."

Mrs. Flander rested, and Ethel tidied the room and piled up some washing.

"Well, my fine family…Ethel and I are going to make our way back into town," Doc said. "Mrs. Flander, I want you to stay in bed for a few days and let your menfolk look after you. Put your babies to your breast. They'll do a lot better that way. Your milk will be in soon."

Doc and Ethel made their way outside into a moonlit night. Driving into town, Ethel saw early signs of Christmas. Coloured candles sat on windowsills, and decorated paper emphasized the store entrances on the main street.

She knew how flickering candles and pretty packages with bows under their Christmas tree would fascinate six-month-old Gordon. He would take great joy in Raymond and Wallace shaking bells and hanging shimmering tinsel.

In the midst of a busy Christmas, Ethel began to make plans for a private maternity hospital in her home—different from the nursing home she'd planned earlier. She applied for appropriate permissions and made necessary arrangements. Her early experience of working in community clinics reinforced the importance of this project.

How many years ago in England had she vowed to continue this work in Canada? She realized it'd never be anything close to Nightingale's in terms of size and numbers, but in love and in time, she'd put her private maternity hospital license on the wall beside her Canadian registered nursing certification. And when that happened, she'd feel that she had carried the torch in her own small way.

chapter twenty-three

Love Finds Its Own

Ethel went into the post office to pick up her mail. A letter from Elsie stuck out from between the envelopes; she could spot that familiar handwriting anywhere. She laid the letter on top of the pile and put the envelopes in her bag. She went straight home, as she always did when a letter came from Elsie. She liked to savour the words without interruption.

Sitting at the kitchen table, she began to read—then she stopped and reread. Standing up, she read the words again, this time aloud:

> "To give you some good news, I have made plans to come to Canada in March. I am very eager to come and be with you, Wallace and the boys. We will have many Christmases together, so I will stay here with the family for this one, and then I'll be able to finish my school year at Easter. I hope this will work well for you. I will send you final plans after the New Year."

Ethel spoke aloud, "It will work well—indeed it will!"

She wiped her eyes again, but this time with tears of joy. What a Christmas present! She could hardly contain her excitement. She walked over to the cupboard and lifted her parents' wedding picture. She traced her finger over their faces. "I'll never forget you. I'll see you on the other side of this life." Ethel was glad they'd written so many letters. Nothing went by that one didn't hurry to share with the other. "There were times when…when I begrudged not having Elsie with me…and resented that you could watch her grow. Forgive me, for I know she was such a blessing to you. You stood in as her mother when I wasn't there, and you gave Elsie the gift of family. Thank you, Mum."

Wallace came striding into the kitchen, his workboots noisily pronouncing each step.

"A letter from Elsie, Wallace. She's coming." Ethel wiped the tears from her eyes as she sat down at the table with her husband. "I can't believe it. Oh, Wallace, will I even know her?"

"Of course you will. You'll know her as much as the day you parted. I'm happy for you."

Several days passed, and although they went about their usual routine, the family had a new sense of purpose.

"There's so much to prepare. I hardly know where to begin," Ethel said.

"Now Ethel," Wallace said, "you've been preparing for more than 10 years for this event. We have a good home to bring Elsie to, and you're still the best cook around. Elsie will get a big welcome from the town. Now, enjoy your Christmas, and when the day comes, we'll all be ready."

Ethel walked over and hugged him. "You're so good for me. I can't begin to tell you how much you settle me in my anxious moments." She pulled her coat off the hook. "I think I'll go for a walk. I need to do some thinking."

Ethel walked down to the church, noticing everything with new eyes: the fences, back stoops and chimneys. She stepped onto the back step of the building and let herself in through the large wooden door. Somebody had just scrubbed the floor and polished the tables—the pine scent still lingered in the air. Ethel walked to the front and sat down on one of the side benches, lowered her head down onto her hands and wept. She pulled Elsie's letter out of her skirt pocket and looked at it. She found it so hard to believe Elsie was coming to…Canada. It was almost too much; she could hardly grasp it.

"Are you all right, Mrs. Bullymore?" Isabelle asked as she slipped onto the bench beside her. "I don't mean to scare you. I saw you come in here, and it ain't Sunday."

"Oh, Isabelle, I didn't even hear you." Ethel wiped away her tears and moved over in the pew. "Yes, I'm all right. Just thinking."

"Are you praying?"

"I should be." Ethel took Isabelle's hand and placed it on one of her own. "But no, I was just thinking."

"Does God hear our thinking?"

"Yes, I'm sure God hears our thoughts before we even put them into words." Ethel opened the letter again. "Here's the evidence of that," she said and wrapped her arms around Isabelle.

Love Finds Its Own

A week later, Ethel picked up the mail to find another letter from Elsie. This one was short: she was to leave March 19th on the SS *Minnedosa* out of Liverpool bound for Saint John, NB and then take the train to Edmonton. It was difficult for Ethel to contain her excitement after she received Elsie's last letter. For that was exactly what it was…her last one.

The town was happy for the Bullymore family. A Christmas party that included the entire community gave everybody a chance to celebrate. Gorton's Hall filled with people talking and laughing, some with hands full of food and others with gifts of celebration.

People quieted when a local storekeeper came to the centre of the crowd. The papers in one hand trembled as he wiped his brow with the other.

"Can I have your attention, folks? This important night dutifully requires somebody to call you to order. Now I'm not much on talking to a large group, but somebody thinks I can do it, so I'll give it my best."

"Let it rip, Will," a voice from the back shouted out, causing a wave of laughter across the room.

"I've been asked to call you to attention and thank you for coming. We also need to thank somebody for all the hard work that she's done, and we're gonna make an announcement of great things to come here in our little town."

Ethel felt all eyes turn towards her. She couldn't believe what she was hearing. What was this, anyway? She stood still and kept her eyes on him as he continued.

"Hank, would you like to take over?"

A tall, lanky rancher from north of Ribstone strolled forward. His big boots resonated on the wooden floor. "Now, what I'm going to say about somebody ain't no surprise to the rest of you. If you was ever in need, you knew you'd be helped. If you got hard of hearing, she'd take the wax out of your ears, or if your sight grew dim, she'd clean your glasses and send you on your way. If you're causing trouble on the main street, she becomes the law. If you're hungry, she becomes the provider. If something needs checkin' about germs and dirt, she becomes the public health officer. If you need to confess or be forgiven, she becomes your priest. If your wife or kids complain about how they're used, she becomes their helpmate. If life's been unkind and you're left feeling like you don't matter, then she finds a way to make you feel like you're '*fearfully and wonderfully made.*' If you're lost, well, her love will shed such a light on you that it'll show you the way home. If you're a different colour, size or religion, then she makes you feel like everybody else. And if you was poor, she'd make you feel like a king. Even the children are not outside her circle of concern. If any try to skip school, she becomes their friendly truant office.

"And a couple more things." Hank smiled sheepishly. "If you get feeling a bit happy from the results of a little too much homebrew, then she'll get on her Johnny-Barleycorn bandwagon and we'll all hear about it. And if you die, well, she might prepare you with your best bib and tucker, lay you out and invite the whole dern town to come have a look at ya."

Everybody laughed. Ethel folded her arms across her chest and laughed with them.

Hank continued, "She's nursed us, buried us, pulled us up by the bootstraps and yes, even at times when necessary, knocked us down at the knees. And it ain't that any of this is easy. I don't know how she makes things happen, but she does; she didn't earn the name Bully for nothin'. We don't have a chance of being any less than what the good Lord made us, or she lets us know. A lot of us are pretty stubborn when it comes to new things. Now, if you take exception to somebody else's behaviour, you'd better have good reason, because she'll call you to account for yourself and want you to ask forgiveness. It's almost easier not to get yourself into trouble than look her in the eye when you're trying to get yourself out of it."

Wallace came up behind Ethel and put his arm around her. Ethel nodded.

Hank went on, "We'd been so used to looking after our own. You know, people come and settle here, make their living, get to know folks, and over time they become part of the community. But she makes us stretch to welcome everybody, immediately. She includes the lost, the loser, the little man, those who don't have nobody to speak for them."

Ethel heard the people turn to one another to talk. Mr. Stoddart from the west concession raised his voice to be heard by the group, "It ain't that she's perfect, because she never was. She don't pretend to be. It's just that she's so dern honest, whether you like it or not, she tells you what you need to hear. And she can be as ornery as anybody else; I've seen it myself, but when it's over, it's over, and she gets on with life." He laughed a hearty laugh, and other folks soon joined in.

Hank held up his hand to quiet the group. "Well, I'm sure you all know who I'm talking about, because you all know why we're here tonight. And that is to honour and show our gratitude. Mrs. Bullymore, would you come up and join me."

Ethel moved slowly towards Hank. She reached up and hugged him. Pulling a corner of his handlebar moustache, she winked at him. "That was quite a speech, Hank. I couldn't imagine who you were talking about until you mentioned those bootstraps." Ethel grinned. "But thank you for those kind words."

"Weren't nothing, ma'am. I didn't have to write it; the missus did that. I only had to read it.

"And something else, ma'am. We know that you've had a letter from England giving you some good news. I understand that in a few months' time, you're going to have just about the most important event ever happen in your life. We want to get a head start on that celebration, because as you get ready to welcome your daughter, you might not have time for us for a little while. We just want to wish you the very best, Mrs. Bullymore."

As she turned around to face her friends, her eyes filled with tears. "I thank you, folks. I too have a grateful heart. I thank you for your best wishes, and I appreciate all of you. I came into your midst as a stranger three years ago. You made me one of your own. Although I loved doing everything I've done, you gave me the opportunity. And so I thank you."

"Wait now, Mrs. Bullymore. We're not through with you yet," Hank continued. "There's something else we got to talk about. Somebody told us, and it was an honest source, that you're going to establish a nursing home there in your house as a private maternity hospital, right? Well, we thought we'd like to give you something to show our appreciation. I mean, we never know when any one of us might end up there."

"Like you said, Hank, it's going to be a private hospital for maternity beds." Ethel raised her eyebrows and looked at her friend. The crowd laughed.

"Yeah, well, I know that, but if any of us needs it, you're not going to turn us away. I know stories of Wallace giving up his bed to make more room for people, even now. So that's already happening."

She smiled. Somebody opening the large front doors caused her to turn her head.

"Come and look out. This is too heavy to bring in."

Ethel walked over to the door and saw a very large box sitting on the landing. Will pulled heavy paper off a beautiful blue corduroy easy chair. Two small boxes rested on the seat.

"For those of you who can't see this gift the men unwrapped, it's a very handsome chair. Is this a hint that I should sit down and enjoy life more?" Ethel laughed.

"Well, maybe. Or it could be that we want you to be comfortable when you do sit down. You know, make it worth your while," Hank said. "And now for these boxes. Open them up so the people can see them."

"These are from the children in the school," one of the parents said. "They know how you always make them feel so important, and they just wanted to give you something back."

Ethel lifted up a small glass globe with a house nestled in willow trees. She smiled as she cradled the paperweight in the palm of her hand.

"Tip it over, Mrs. Bullymore. Turn it over," a child's voice raised over the noise of the room.

Small white snow particles fell over the house as Ethel turned it in her hand.

A woman's voice carried across the room. "It's a picture of peace, even in a snowstorm."

"And here's the other gift, Ethel," Hank said.

Ethel removed a small black leather case from its package. "It's a thermometer. Thank you. I will treasure it."

"You see, that's the hint for you to keep working. We can't have you sitting in that easy chair too much, playing with your paperweight."

"Speech! Speech!" Voices bantered back and forth.

"I thank you so much. It's good to be in a large family such as all of you have provided. I came to this town filled with grief, and your love kept healing me in many ways. I look forward to continue working in your midst. I hope I don't have to lay too many of you out; I'd rather pull you up by the bootstraps."

The people laughed as that image formed in their minds, and they nodded their heads.

"In all seriousness, I think we agree that the health and welfare of the town and districts are better when people help people. When we work together, we all benefit. Thank you again."

Wallace came and stood beside Ethel, and the crowd applauded. She was filled with gratitude for the people as she continued to mix with them. Later, when Gordon began to fret and Raymond appeared tired, she and Wallace gathered them up, and they left for home.

The oil lamps lit the way as they walked out with others. Some folks walked to cars parked on the street. Others walked to the livery stable where they had left their horses. A few walked down the roads to their homes, while the snow fell softly on the branches of leafless trees.

"Strange, isn't it," Ethel said softly to Wallace as they turned toward their house, "how things are sometimes prepared for us to do; it just takes us a little time to get around to them. It seems that town gatherings give opportunity for things to happen and unite people at the same time. Their love and need to care for one another brings them together, and then God blesses them even more."

Christmas came with all its lights, decorations and presents. It was a joyous time. Ethel couldn't help but think of the many Christmas trees they'd decorated without Elsie, but she knew that next year would be different. She had new feelings of anticipation. However, as much as she wanted Elsie with her, she was rightfully spending this last Christmas with the family in England.

On New Year's Day, Wallace came home from the Cozy Café with the sad news that one of the children from the South School District was missing. The boy hadn't shown up for breakfast with the rest of the family, and they thought he might have slipped out during the night. When they were looking for him, they found a package with Christmas cake crumbs and some crusts in the root cellar.

"What on earth would he be doing in the root cellar?" Ethel asked.

"Nobody knows."

"Which one of the boys was it?"

"Joe, Bud and Bessie's second oldest."

Ethel remembered Joe as a likable boy—not a troublemaker or trickster. "Had he been punished or disciplined?" Ethel poised the question that could give them some clues.

"Yes," Wallace said, stroking his chin thoughtfully. "Apparently he'd been checked, but not to the extent that he'd have run away because of it. Children have to be able to take discipline."

"I agree, but sometimes they're acting out at something totally different than what parents think. It's like walking past somebody at night and not being aware of them."

"Well, for whatever reason it happened, it's too cold outside for a ten-year-old to be away from the warmth of his home."

"Or the love of his family, especially if he's upset about something. That's two things he's coping with: his first issue unknown to anybody, and then his parents' reprimand—even deserved, nonetheless felt."

Ethel's heart was troubled for the youngster, and she wished she could help. She remembered him well—brown curly hair and a captivating smile; his mother and father must be worrying. Ethel couldn't imagine if it were Raymond; even at the thought of this, her pulse quickened.

"I'm going with some of the other fathers to visit a few of the farms around," Wallace said. "I can't see him walking any distance. The snow's not deep, but it was too cold last night to go far on foot. I wonder if they checked to see if his pony was gone. Remember we used to see that boy riding across the hills south of town, as if the Great Spirit and all his warriors were chasing him."

"I remember." Ethel smiled. "I'm so glad you're going, Wallace. They'll need everybody they can get, and time is important because of this weather."

"We'll find him. Like I say, he can't be too far."

"I wonder," Ethel said, "if he's over at his grandpa's house. Didn't we hear at the party that his grandfather wasn't expected to see Christmas?"

"You're right. They probably wouldn't tell the old folks about the boy being missing, not wanting to worry them, so they may not have thought to go over there and check."

"I think we're on to something," Ethel said.

"And the boy wouldn't know about his grandpa possibly dying. They wouldn't have told him."

"Don't underestimate a child. They have heart language when it comes to grandparents," Ethel said. "When you go out looking, check to see if the pony's in the barn, and then go to the grandpa's house. That boy's a good lad. He's had nothing to run away for, but he might think he had something to run to."

During Wallace's absence, Ethel offered a word of prayer. Separation from a child was a heartbreaking experience. Even the shock that he was not there at breakfast would have frightened the family. Ethel knew the search would be thorough as the men looked through the buildings and talked to neighbours and friends.

Children—what a gift, a responsibility and a challenge. Elsie's first four years were indelibly etched in Ethel's mind and so deeply ingrained they had fed the last 10 years with memories. The reality of their reunion continued to bring a wave of tears to her eyes. She could not bear to think of losing a child.

She thought of another boy, Tommy, and his parents. He'd died a while back, and she wondered how they were faring. She must visit them soon. Nothing grieves a community more than the death of a child. And now, a missing one.

Later that day, Wallace came in with a wide smile. "We were right: the pony and the grandparents. The sorrow that lad felt after his scolding had fed the sorrow he was already feeling about his grandpa being sick. He packed some food; looked like he ate it while getting warm in the barn, probably after he saddled his pony. It's good he didn't have far to go and pretty smart of him to go on horseback. Anyway, the outside door of the back porch was open, and he went straight to his grandpa's room and lay down beside him."

"Leave it to children, eh?" Ethel smiled. "They know how to grieve better than any of us; no pretence, just reality."

"And that's not all, Ethel. His grandpa died this afternoon. The parents found him when they went in to check."

Ethel just looked at Wallace. Tears brimmed her eyes. "Isn't that something? Wouldn't it be like standing on holy ground to listen to their last conversation?"

During a snowstorm that seemed to come out of nowhere, Ethel conceded to pulling the heavy curtains to hide the frosted windows and putting towels along the bottom of both outside doors. Thank goodness for that leftover stew and freshly baked bread—at least she didn't have to prepare a big supper. Both Wallace and Gordon had curled up on the chesterfield, and Raymond was playing with his new wheels Wallace had carved for him. She had some time to herself.

Ethel's journal lay on the edge of her sewing basket, drawing her attention to the fact she hadn't continued to write as she'd promised herself. After reaching for it, she picked it up and laid it open on the table. Picking up her pencil, she began:

> I remember with affection Edie and George Buchanan living at the edge of town. They've always been supportive of my work and told me about the man, I never did write his name down, who brought his wife to their house in a sleigh. When they opened the door, the man hollered, "We can't get any further. Can you go get Bully and bring her out? Maw's on a blanket in the back of the sleigh."

> Edie told me about another time when a young girl appeared at their door after walking in from the country. "I just can't go any further," she'd said. "I'm too cold." Edie had asked her, "What on earth would you have done if nobody'd been home here?" There was no hesitation in the girl's voice. "I guess I'd of had to try to get into town and go to Mrs. Bullymore's house."

> And then there was the situation when a woman crept to the house from her sleigh through five-foot-high snowdrifts. I had to go out into

the yard to help her, and not long after we got her into the house, I delivered her baby.

And the woman who walked with her husband from their house to our front door. The snow was deep and her legs weren't long enough to step over the banks. The woman, already in intense labour, got stuck. Between me, Wallace, and the woman's husband, we got her into the house on time—but not by much.

I remember some of the most difficult situations of bringing new life into the world when farmers had to do a sophisticated relay work in the midst of violent winter storms. "I can only get Ma so far; you'll have to take her the rest of the way." They'd move the couch from one sleigh to another with the woman hanging on and praying she'd arrive at our house safely.

Even though their goals were the same, "bring that baby into the world and keep Ma safe," every story was different in its own way.

I would be amiss if I didn't make note of the time when Wallace carefully built a small wooden casket and I folded a remnant of silk around the inside corners. Surely, the words said at this time were comforting.

And there was always room for another baby. When we ran out of crib space, the top drawer of the dresser opened nicely to provide a perfect-sized bed for a newborn.

Closing the journal, she laid her pencil down, giving thanks for those who had come to mind. There would be more stories when there was time to write them down.

PART IV
1921

chapter twenty-four

Elsie Comes Home

The Christmas festivities filtered into January. People gathered at the town hall for their games and music nights. The churches planned ongoing suppers and dramas. Several wedding groups had parties in Gorton's Hall. Both Wallace and Ethel played their share of curling. The weather stayed fine, with only a few bad storms to hinder travel. February slipped away, and March came with anticipation of Elsie's arrival.

Ethel awakened at 4 a.m. on that long-awaited day. Her thoughts tumbled through her mind: feelings of doubt, fear, anxiety and euphoric joy. *This is the day…the day that Elsie comes,* kept circling in her mind.

Was she ready? Would she meet Elsie's approval? Whatever would Elsie think of their town? Never mind that—what about the family? *Thank goodness for letters; at least we're not total strangers to her.* Yet, even though Ethel'd constantly thought about it since she received Elsie's last letter, her arrival still didn't seem real. In the past there was always something that had hindered her passage, but today she would see her daughter. "My Elsie, a young woman now. Will I even know her?"

Ethel got up, washed, made the porridge and boiled the kettle. She dressed in her favourite wool skirt and hand-knit sweater, finished her preparations and finally sat down to savour her tea. She thought back over the past years; the quiet house seemed to honour her thoughts. The last time she'd seen Elsie she was sitting in her grandmother's arms, waving a white handkerchief, pretending she was on the Liverpool dock. In those early years, not a day had passed that Ethel hadn't thought of her, hadn't prayed that if she couldn't come that year, then maybe the next year.

After Wallace and the boys had eaten their breakfast, they said their goodbyes, promising to be on the platform when she and Elsie arrived.

At 8 o'clock sharp, Ethel boarded the train for her long trip to Edmonton. She looked at her watch every few minutes. She tried to doze, but her mind filled with words and images. She brought out her stationery that she'd carried to write some letters, but she ruined every sheet with scribbles and drawings. Words of prayer seem to fade into the garble of conversation rising above the seats. Continual movement and occasional swaying coaxed Ethel into moments of inner peace, only to have raised voices or crying children snatch it away. Out of the window, she watched the train's shadow charge across the flat prairie land that lay ready to waken after a long winter's slumber, and then she closed her eyes to think. Suddenly, the train decreased speed. Ethel checked her watch: 11:15 a.m. She only had about 40 minutes before Elsie's train was due in Edmonton from Montreal.

After what seemed like an eternity, the appointed time arrived. Ethel hurried from one train to the other and stood at the gate, waiting, watching for Elsie.

At high noon, right on schedule, the black locomotive arrived, emerging through its own smoke as it chugged into the station. Ethel waited and watched every window for a white glove. She wondered how her daughter, raised in English etiquette, would adapt to the West, especially in the cold month of March.

She saw several people file down the steps of the train and glance over the crowd and then wave and smile, having found a known face. Suddenly, there appeared before her the anxious face of her daughter: yes, just like her picture, beautiful and graceful as she moved onto the station platform. An ankle-length brown skirt topped stylish boots, and a fashionable woollen coat with a fur collar fit neatly over her youthful body. Her dark eyes, set over flushed cheeks, scanned the crowd.

Ethel waved and waved. She stood on her tiptoes and frantically flailed her arms, but Elsie seemed to look past her, gleaning the crowd as if looking for a familiar face. A look of urgency shadowed her eyes as she brushed away a wisp of dark-brown hair.

Ethel could wait no longer. Tears flowed down her cheeks as she ran towards Elsie, bumping and pushing people, unapologetically rushing forward. Moving through the crowd, she gathered her skirts and ascended the stairs. There on the platform she quickly embraced her daughter. Arms that had yearned for so many years to feel the warmth of her baby now wrapped tightly around Elsie.

Ethel's voice choked in the tension of the moment. "Elsie, Elsie! My little girl all grown up. Oh, my precious one, I just want to hold you."

"Mummy, is this you...really you?" Elsie wept. She stood as tall as Ethel and cupped Ethel's face in her hands. "How I've dreamt of this moment so many times, only to wake up and find you not with me."

Tender hugs and words consumed the next few moments. They cried openly and wiped tears from each other's eyes.

"Come, let me look at you. You're all grown up and, I must say, a very lovely young lady." Ethel touched her face.

"And you're just as I knew you'd be," Elsie said softly. "Here, I brought you something that Gran kept for me. She said I was to give it to you the minute I saw you."

Elsie placed a white hankie in Ethel's hand. "I was told to wave it hard the day you left. I waved it for many years after that day and pretended you were coming back. Gran said that this'd be the last thing you'd remember when you left our house and the first thing you'd think of when you boarded the ship."

"I remember, dear. Oh, how I remember that hankie. Thank you. Come on home now; it's been a long trip, and you must be dreadfully tired."

"Yes, I am, but I just want to talk to you. I have so much to tell you and so many questions to ask. Anyway, I'm too excited to rest," Elsie replied.

"I can only imagine; I know what it's like for me." Ethel smiled. "After we depart, we still have another three-hour train ride ahead of us. It will be a wonderful time for us to talk about so many things. Then when we get to Edgerton, you'll meet the family. They've been looking forward to welcoming you into the community. After that, of all things, we have a party to attend."

Ethel and Elsie climbed the steps into the passenger car of the train that would take them home. They talked, rested and talked some more. They sat side by side, holding each other's hands, then folding them in their laps, only to reach out for each other again as they chatted and laughed and cried.

"We'll come back into Edmonton when the weather gets nice. I'll take you to the place where your pa and I lived. And we'll go to Beechmount Cemetery where he's laid to rest."

"I'm sorry life didn't work out for you over here as you and Pa planned."

"I am too, but he had some very good years after he left England. For that, I am grateful. He always looked forward to the time when you might be able to come. He waited for your letters and cherished your pictures. Oh, I've so much to tell you about him and some pictures to show you too. However, we've a lifetime ahead of us, my dear. Now tell me about your grandmother and your grandfather."

Elsie's facial expression saddened at the change in subject, but she quickly brightened and continued to chat.

"They talked about you every day, Mummy. It was like you could be coming over for supper anytime. Gran made it seem like you were close by. They loved you, wanted you, but at the same time they knew your place was here in Canada doing what you had to do."

"I'm sorry I couldn't be of help in those last days."

"It was hard on everybody when they died so close together. But that was like them in life too. What one did, the other did. Gran didn't suffer. Aunt Mabel was there a lot, and others too. At the end, she had a hard time breathing and she slept a lot, and then one day…she just didn't wake up."

"And the funeral? Tell me more," Ethel asked. "Was it pleasant? Did Mum look nice?"

"Yes, she did, and everybody came home, even my cousins from Scotland. We had the service in the church. Yes, it was just like Gran wanted it. And Grandad, he looked so young when he was laid out—even his wrinkles disappeared."

Ethel laughed and thanked Elsie for making it real for her. She told her daughter about life in the West and about the family in Edgerton and how excited Wallace and Raymond were to meet her and that they'd been telling little Gordon all about her even though he was still young. She described their home, the church and the neighbourhood to Elsie. Time went quickly, and soon they were pulling into Edgerton's station.

Ethel and Elsie held hands and grinned at each other as they stood in the aisle between the seats waiting for the train to stop. "If I don't settle down, they'll be taking me off here on a stretcher." Ethel's heart beat so loudly she thought it'd explode.

"I know what you mean, Mummy. I'm so excited. I'm finally here and with you." She reached over again and hugged her mother. "I feel that I should pinch myself to see if I'm dreaming."

The black locomotive chugged into the station. As it crept to a stop, images of faces, waving hands and flying flags filled the view. Familiar scenes flashed by the windows as Ethel peered out. People filled the platform and leaned against the fence. *My goodness, the whole town has come.*

"There's a crowd out there," Ethel said. "Are you ready for this, Elsie? People are used to coming and sitting on the platform even on cold days. They like to see the local train go through with all its smoke and fury, but I think everybody and their cousins have turned out today."

"I've been waiting a long time to come. If I can do it as well as I've practiced over the years, I'll be fine." Elsie laughed, her cheeks turning pink at the admission.

Ethel led the way out onto the platform; then Elsie joined her and they stood there together, hand in hand.

A group of people faced them, wiping their eyes and smiling through their tears. Friends from the community, farmers from the country, even the station attendants cheered and applauded.

Turning from the crowd, Ethel said to Elsie, "These are our friends and family and soon to be yours."

Wallace shifted little Gordon on one hip and walked towards Ethel and Elsie, while holding Raymond's hand. He handed Gordon to his mother and then put his arms around Elsie and gave her a hug. "Welcome, Elsie. You've made your mother very happy and the rest of us too. We're all so glad you've come home."

An elderly man leaned over and spoke softly to Elsie. "We're real glad to have you with us, Miss Elsie. We hope you'll be happy here." He handed her a small sheaf of flowers with a velvet bow, covered with cellophane to protect them from the cold air.

Elsie placed them in her arms and said, "I hope so too. It seems in my mind that I've been coming forever. Thank you so much for the flowers."

The man turned toward the eager crowd. "Okay, folks, it's cold out here. Remember, you're all invited over to Gorton's Hall for a potluck supper at six o'clock to meet Miss Elsie Ayres and to wish her well in Canada."

Ethel knew her family had now taken a different shape; they were changed. As they walked home, she felt a sense of pride. Life would be more complete than it had ever been before. She delighted in the fact that her loved ones were together in this place. There'd still be letters to England for her remaining family, but she finally experienced a natural closure to the past.

As a family, they spent precious time in the privacy of their home, sharing pictures, reminiscing and talking about the future. Ethel didn't want separation from Elsie even for a moment, but she knew the girl was exhausted, so she showed Elsie her room and encouraged her to lie down for a brief rest before the evening meal. Ethel had dreamt of this day for so long and had even practiced how she'd take her to the bedroom. It was a pretty room with fresh wallpaper of fashionable colours. Matching fabric covered the chairs, and a petite porcelain doll sat on a matching footstool. A long mirror, with a beautiful casing crafted by Wallace's hands, stood against the wall. And the bed looked warm and inviting with its feather-tick mattress and big pillows.

Ethel looked in on Elsie later and found her sound asleep. A doll lay in the crook of her arm—the same doll Ethel had packed everywhere they went when Elsie was a child. She didn't want to wake her, but she knew the town was expecting them at the reception.

Ethel bent over to touch Elsie's shoulder and noticed a handkerchief that had fallen from her hand. She picked it up. It was moist. Ethel looked closer at Elsie and knew she'd been crying.

"Elsie dear, can you wake up?" Ethel asked gently. She nudged her shoulder a little.

Elsie opened her eyes and smiled at Ethel. "Is it time to go?"

"It is, dear." Ethel paused. "Is everything all right? I mean…were you crying?"

Elsie sighed. "It's just all so different. I feel so strange. I thought it would be—"

"I'm sorry, Elsie. We'll try to make it as easy as we can for you. Is there anything you'd like to talk about?"

She hesitated. "When I was a little girl, I wondered why you left me behind in England. Over the years, Gran told me the reason again and again. She told me you loved me so much you didn't want to risk my health in a strange country when I was sickly. I tried hard to remember you—your face and your voice. I asked Gran many times what you were doing, where you were going and who your friends were. She told me about my father, and I got to know his family a little bit. I liked them a lot. But when I got your letter and you said Pa had died, I couldn't believe it. It wasn't fair. And now that I'm here with you, I keep thinking he…he should be here too. He got cheated, and I did too." Elsie started to cry and covered her face in the pillow.

"I don't know what to say, dear. I loved your pa very much and felt terribly alone when he died. It was a long time before I could go on in life without him." Ethel stroked her daughter's hair and sat in silence for a few seconds before saying, "I'm sorry that I didn't prepare you better for missing him when you came. I want you to feel at home with us, but I know how important your memories of your pa are."

Elsie didn't say anything. She just lay there looking straight ahead. Every once in a while, her body shuddered as if it were being dragged over rough ground. Ethel wanted to make everything right for her. She wanted to take away her pain and give her a sense of closure. But in her mind, this grand accomplishment of Elsie coming to Canada…to Edgerton…to Ethel was obviously not completion for her but one more loss in a childhood of sorrow. Only honouring this would bring healing, and help her to accept new life here.

"And I miss Gran and my young aunties and all my friends." Elsie began to sob again and wiped her eyelids with the handkerchief. "Oh, I miss Gran so much."

Waves of helplessness consumed Ethel. She had focused so much on herself that she'd somehow missed Elsie's burden of loneliness and the sorrow she would feel for what she'd left behind. Ethel reached over and drew Elsie near, and they both wept.

"I'm very sorry, luv. You have given up so much. We'll try together. And we won't forget that this is not all about reunion; it's about remembering our past, too."

Elsie blew her nose, reached for a dry handkerchief and wiped her eyes. "Thank you, Mummy." She looked at Ethel and leaned over to hug her again. "Thank you for listening. I shouldn't have blathered like that, but I just couldn't go to the party without telling you; I knew you'd understand."

"I'm learning, dear. My goodness, I'd have missed something special had you not told me."

"And there's something else I've worried about." Elsie paused. "What must the people think of me not coming to Canada before this?"

"Why, they understand, dear. They know you couldn't leave England because of your health until we got established in Edmonton." Ethel wiped a tear from Elsie's cheek. "And then the war and the influenza. Your grandparents' health and getting everything settled and sorted afterwards…oh, there were so many reasons."

"But I didn't know how to come or even if I really wanted to come. Because all I knew was Enfield and the family there."

"They won't have thought about all of that. Don't you worry. They will love you because I love you." Ethel hesitated and took a deep breath. "Would you like to come down now? We've a party to go to…for you."

"Yes, Mummy. I want to go to my party," Elsie said. "I'm very happy to be here, truly I am."

"I know, dear," Ethel said. "And I'm happy you're here."

Later when they walked into Gorton's Hall, people cheered and applauded. Residents of the town filled the room to overflowing. Balloons hung from the ceiling of the old hall, adding a festive touch. Ribbons and bows of complementary colours dangled from the posts. The family moved graciously from one person to another, greeting and introducing Elsie.

"The room is so beautiful," Elsie said.

"Yes, indeed. And you will find the people likewise, dear," Ethel said.

Ethel watched the town open its heart again and accept one whom they had grown to love over the last few years but had never met—until tonight. Ethel shared her life with such a wise and loving husband and, now, three wonderful children. She looked around at her friends, remembering that she had come here as a stranger and had been taught the ways of the community by caring people.

She'd learned a valuable lesson. When life dumped problems into her lap, God gave her all the tools she needed to sort through them. For that, she was so thankful.

She knew that not everything had happened as planned, but most things had worked together for good. She had continued to live out her dream expectantly until it turned around to face her and became a reality.

Nurse Rankin's words that labour pains were a prelude to new life filtered through her mind. Ethel reflected on the past 10 years, grateful for all the people and experiences she had known, and she gave thanks for the day and all it held.

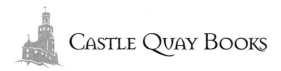

OTHER AWARD WINNING CASTLE QUAY TITLES INCLUDE:
Bent Hope (Tim Huff)
The Beautiful Disappointment (Colin McCartney)
The Cardboard Shack Beneath the Bridge (Tim Huff)
Certainty (Grant Richison) - NEW!
Dancing with Dynamite (Tim Huff) - NEW! 2011 Book of the Year Award!
Deciding to Know God in a Deeper Way (Sam Tita) - NEW!
The Defilers (Deborah Gyapong)
Father to the Fatherless (Paul Boge)
Find a Broken Wall (Brian Stiller) - NEW!
Hope for the Hopeless (Paul Boge) - NEW!
I Sat Where They Sat (Arnold Bowler)
Jesus and Caesar (Brian Stiller)
Keep On Standing (Darlene Polachic)
The Kingdom Promise (Gary Gradley & Phil Kershaw)
The Leadership Edge (Elaine Stewart-Rhude)
Leaving a Legacy (David C. Bentall) - NEW!
Making Your Dreams Your Destiny (Judy Rushfeldt)
Mentoring Wisdom (Dr. Carson Pue) - NEW!
Mere Christian (Michael Coren)
Mormon Crisis (James Beverley)
One Smooth Stone (Marcia Lee Laycock)
Our Father: the Prodigal Son Returns (Pastor Bruce Smith & Phil Kershaw)
Predators Live Among Us: Protect Your Family from Child Sex Abuse
(Diane Roblin-Lee) - NEW!
Red Letter Revolution (Colin McCartney)
Reflections (Cal Bombay) - NEW!
Seven Angels for Seven Days (Angelina Fast-Vlaar)
Stop Preaching and Start Communicating (Tony Gentilucci) - NEW!
Through Fire & Sea (Marilyn Meyers)
To My Family (Diane Roblin-Lee)
Vision that Works (David Collins)
Walking Towards Hope (Paul Boge)
What Happens When I Die (Brian Stiller) - NEW!
The Way They Should Go (Kirsten Femson)
You Never Know What You Have Till You Give It Away (Brian Stiller)

For a full list of all Castle Quay and BayRidge book titles visit
www.castlequaybooks.com